EASY MEMORY GAMES & PUZZLES

Includes Relaxing Memory Activities and Fun Classic Puzzles

BY JOY KINNEST

LOMIC BOOKS

EASY MEMORY GAMES & PUZZLES

Includes Relaxing Memory Activities and Fun Classic Puzzles

By Joy Kinnest

ISBN: 978-1-988923-55-0

Published by Lomic Books
Kitchener, Ontario

Copyright

Disclaimer

The puzzles and games in this book are for entertainment purposes only. Although the author and publisher have worked hard to ensure that the information in this book is accurate, the reader should be aware that errors or omissions may occur. The author and publisher disclaim any liability to any person or party for any loss resulting from reliance on any information in this book.

CONTENTS

CONTENTS CONTINUED

Section One

MEMORY GAMES

FIND THE PICTURE

HOW TO PLAY

Find the Picture

1. Memorize the item.

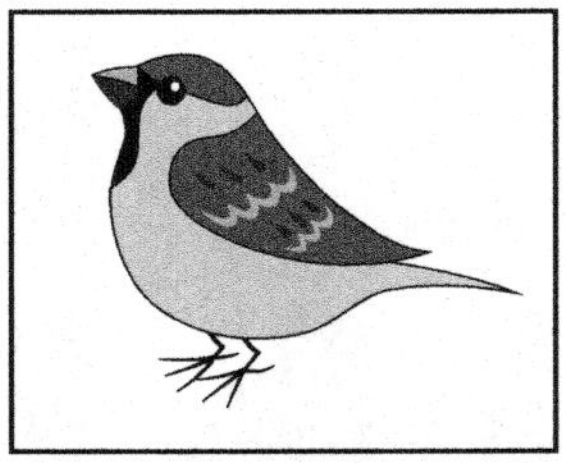

2. Turn the page.

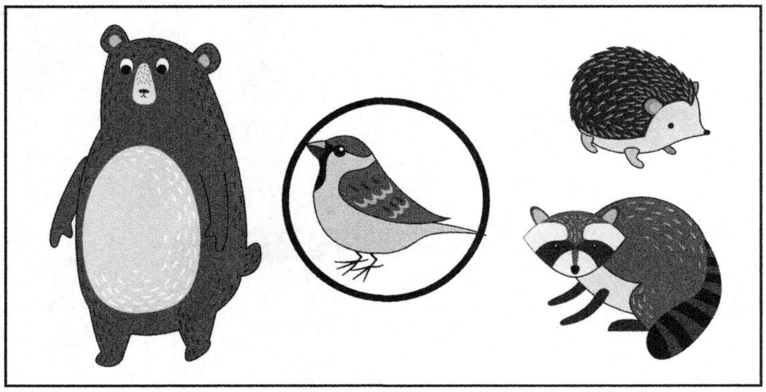

3. Circle the item you remember.

Helpful Hints!

✓ You only need to memorize what the item is, not the details of the picture. In the example above, the picture is of a bird. So, you just need to remember "bird," not any of the details found in the drawing.

✓ Take your time memorizing the item, there is no rush. Also, feel free to try each memory game as many times as you would like.

Find the Picture

Picture One:

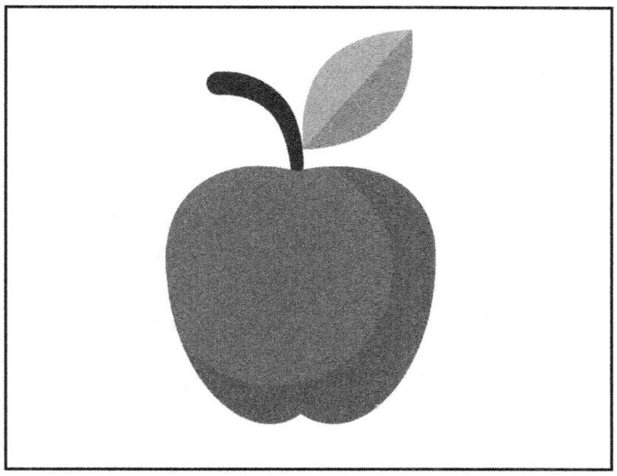

Memorize the item above. Then turn the page, and circle the item you memorized.

turn the page

Picture Two:

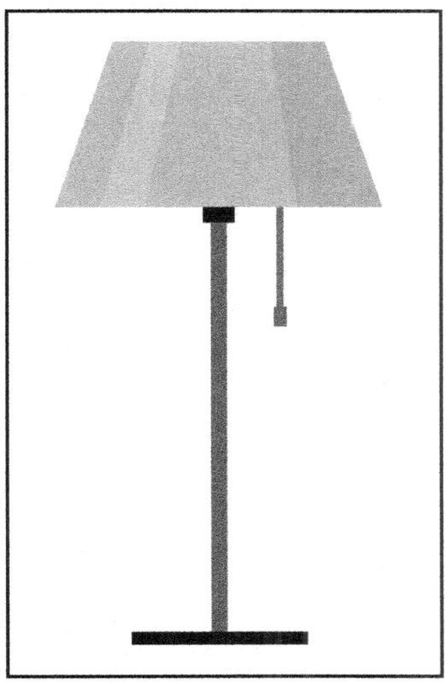

Memorize the item above. Then turn the page, and circle the item you memorized.

turn the page

Memory Game

Puzzle continued from the previous page.

Picture One

Circle the item you memorized.

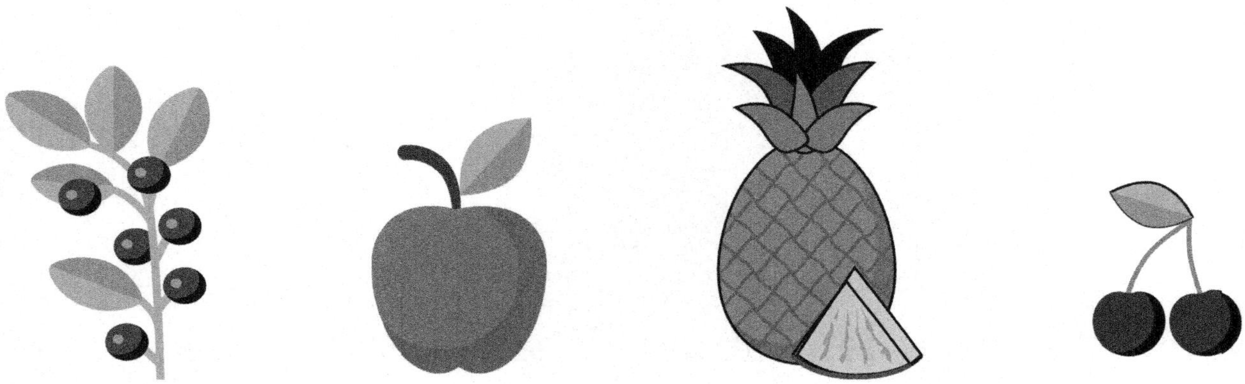

Picture Two

Circle the item you memorized.

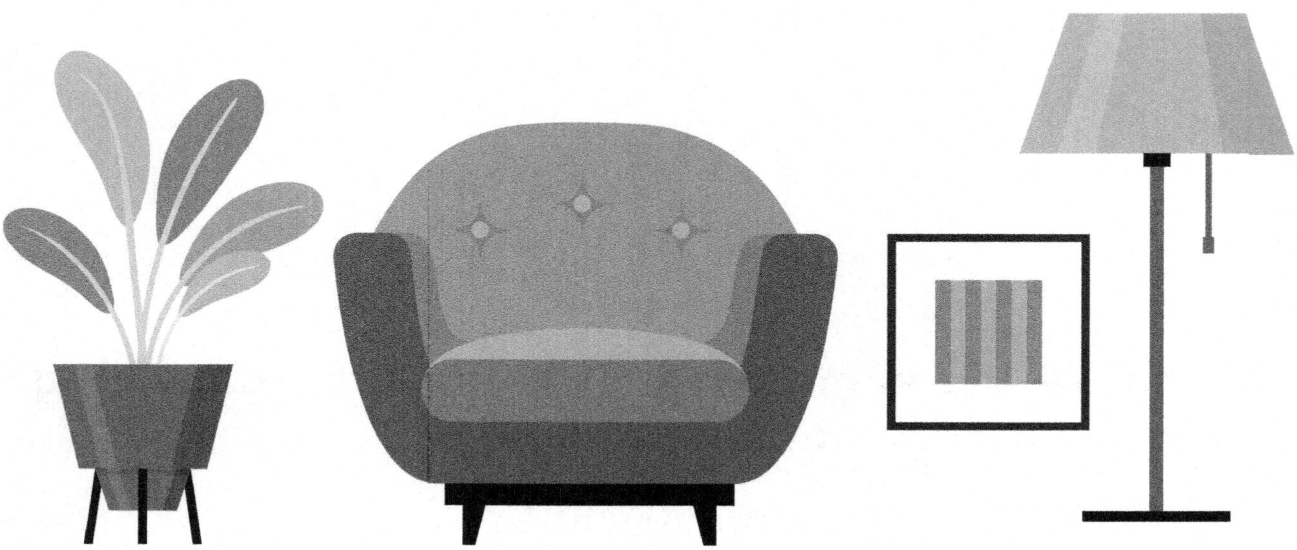

Find the Picture

Picture One:

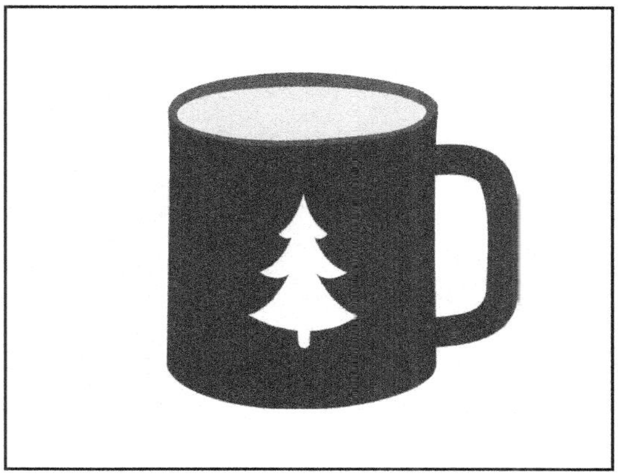

Memorize the item above. Then turn the page, and circle the item you memorized.

turn the page

Picture Two:

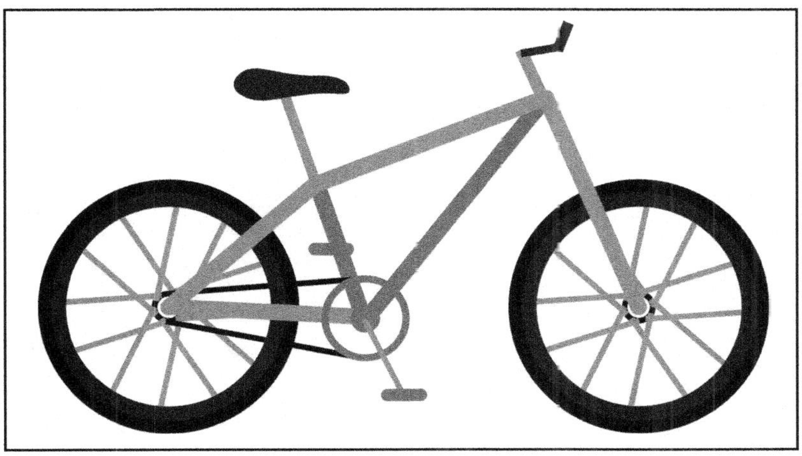

Memorize the item above. Then turn the page, and circle the item you memorized.

turn the page

Memory Game

Puzzle continued from the previous page.

Picture One

Circle the item you memorized.

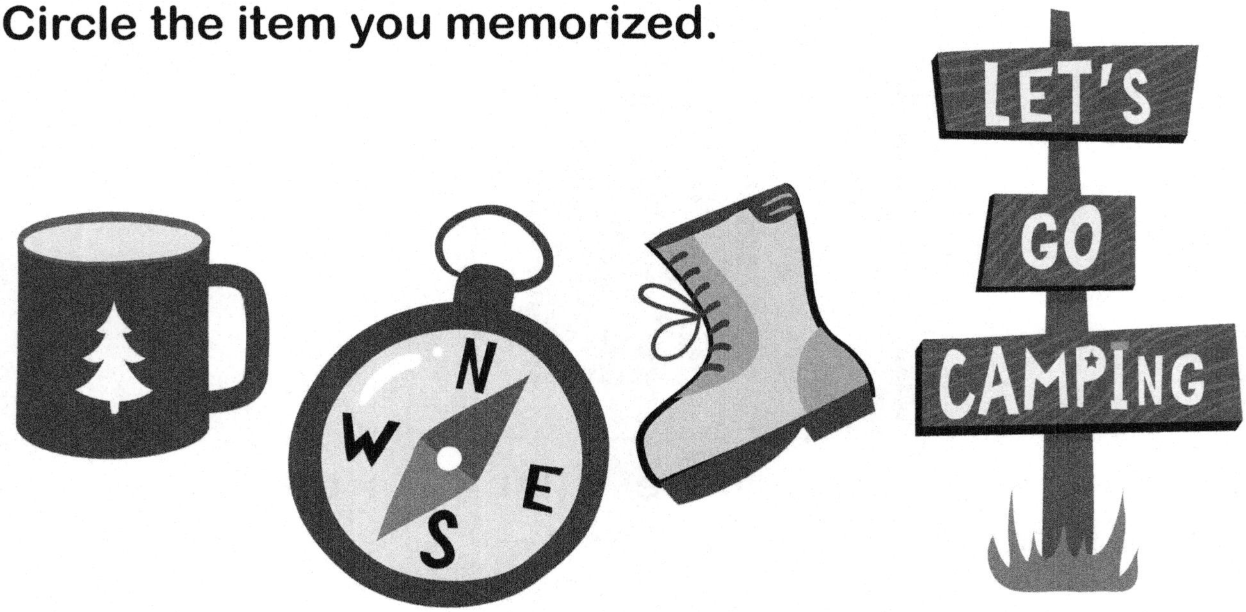

Picture Two

Circle the item you memorized.

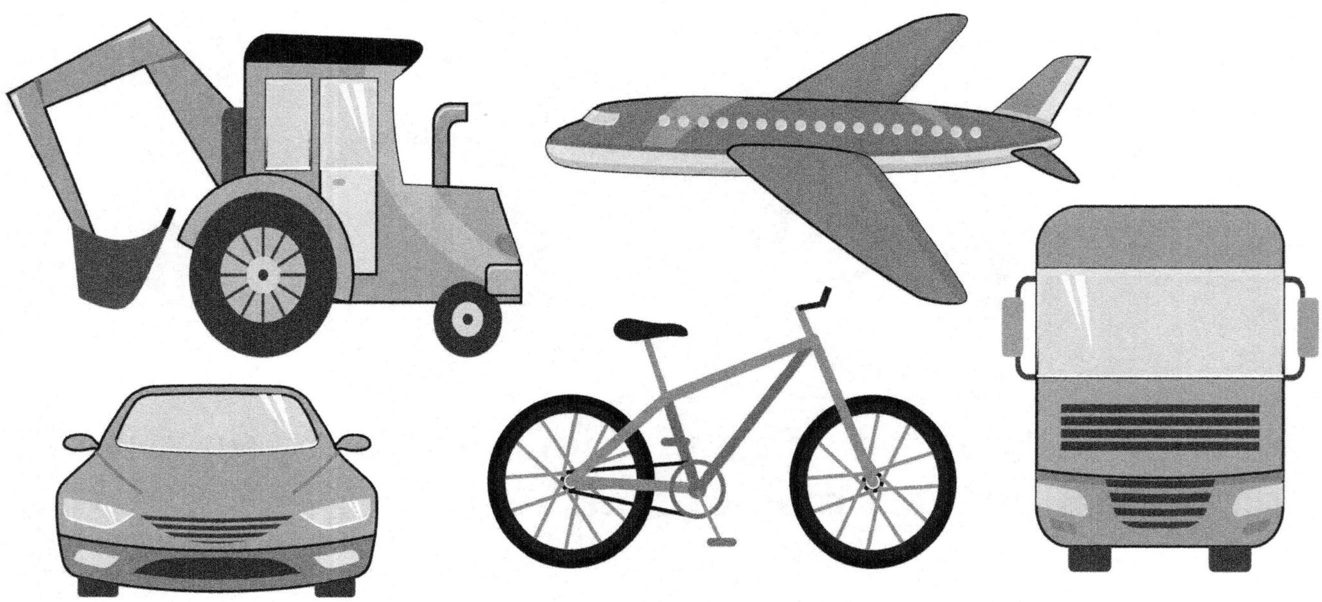

Find the Picture

Picture One:

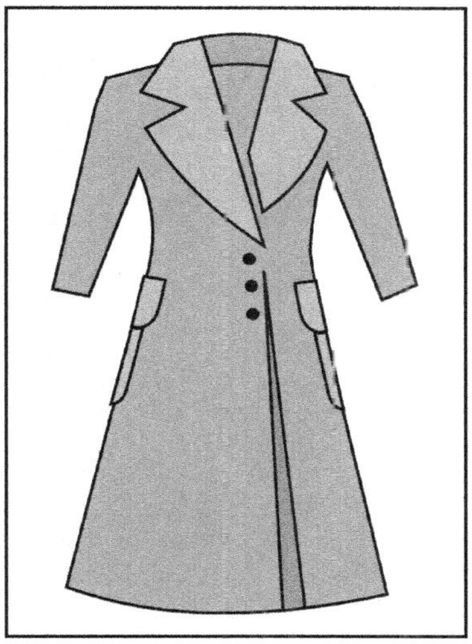

Memorize the item above. Then turn the page, and circle the item you memorized.

turn the page

Picture Two:

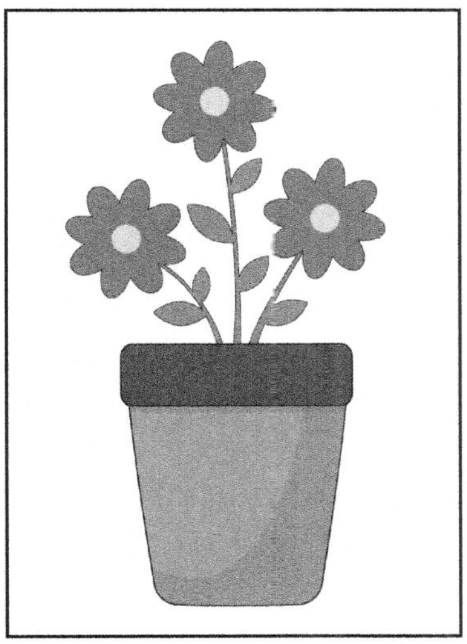

Memorize the item above. Then turn the page, and circle the item you memorized.

turn the page

Puzzle continued from the previous page.

Picture One

Circle the item you memorized.

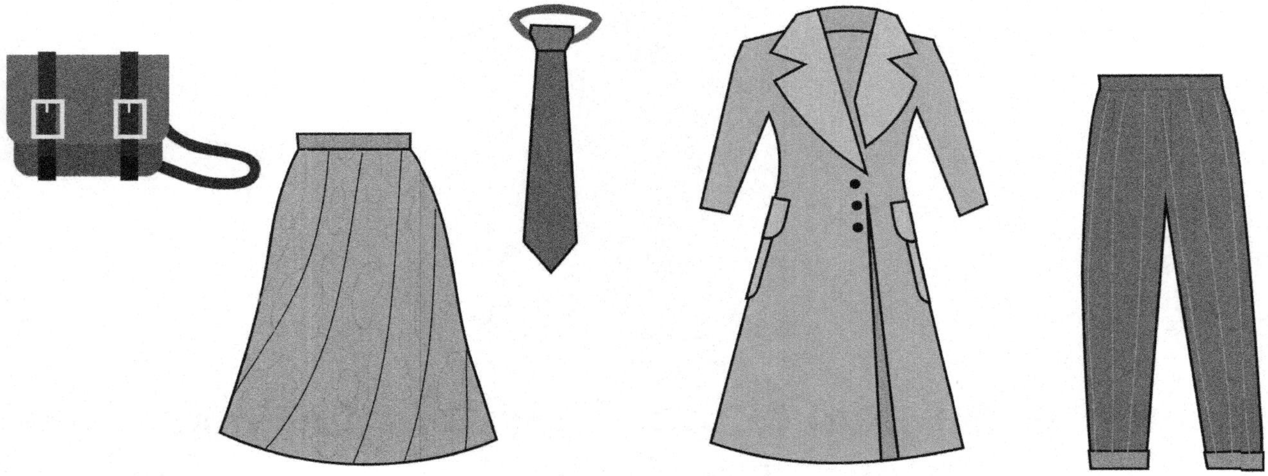

Picture Two

Circle the item you memorized.

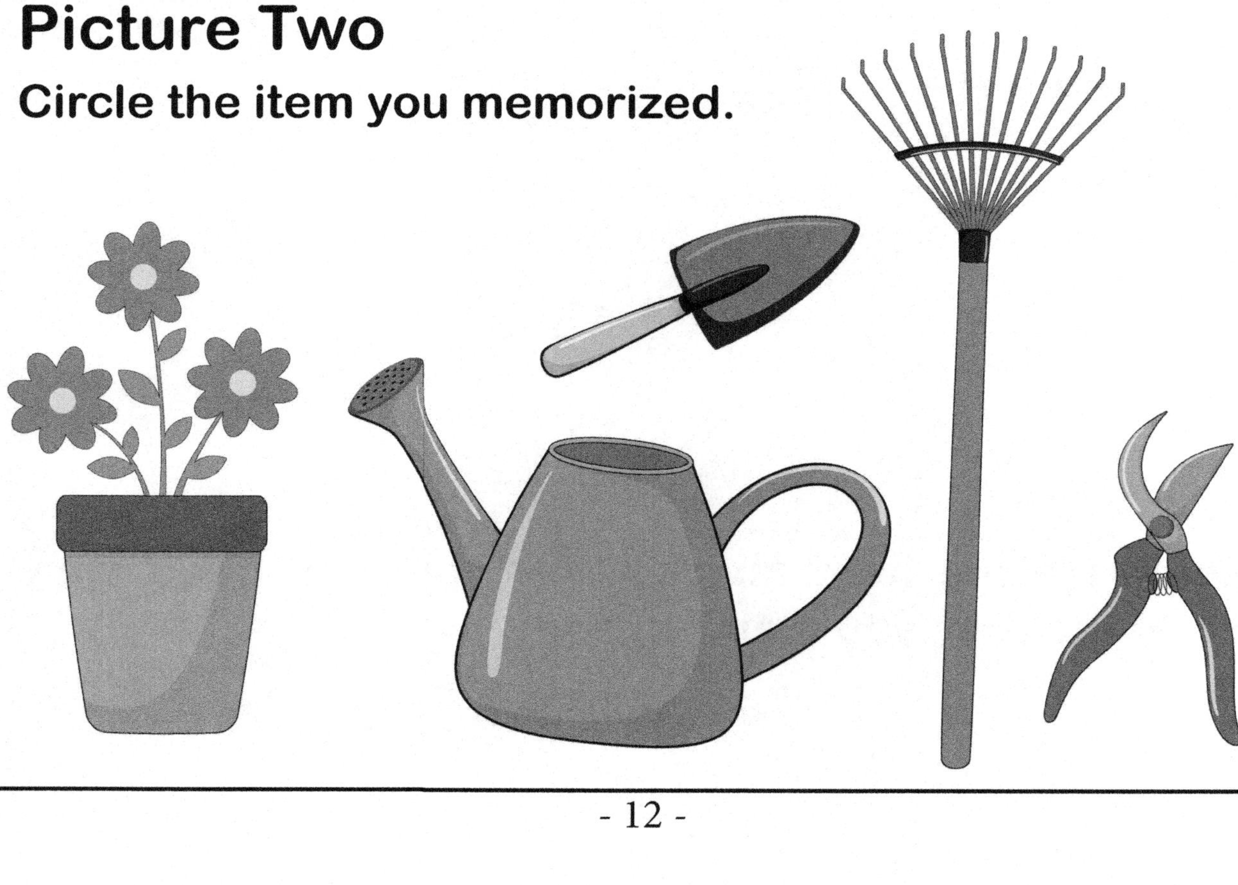

Find the Picture

Picture One:

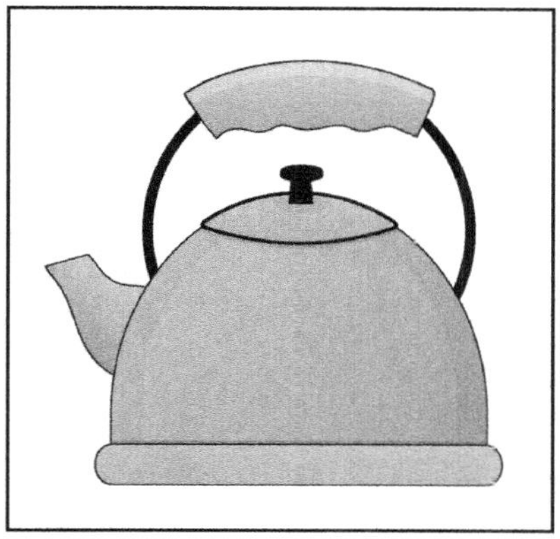

Memorize the item above. Then turn the page, and circle the item you memorized.

turn the page

Picture Two:

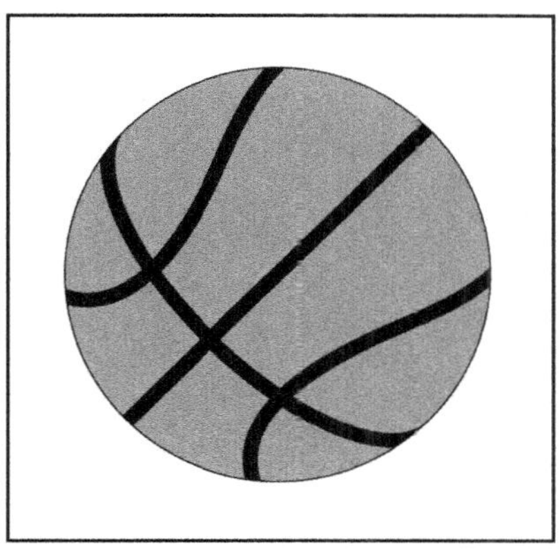

Memorize the item above. Then turn the page, and circle the item you memorized.

turn the page

Memory Game

Puzzle continued from the previous page.

Picture One

Circle the item you memorized.

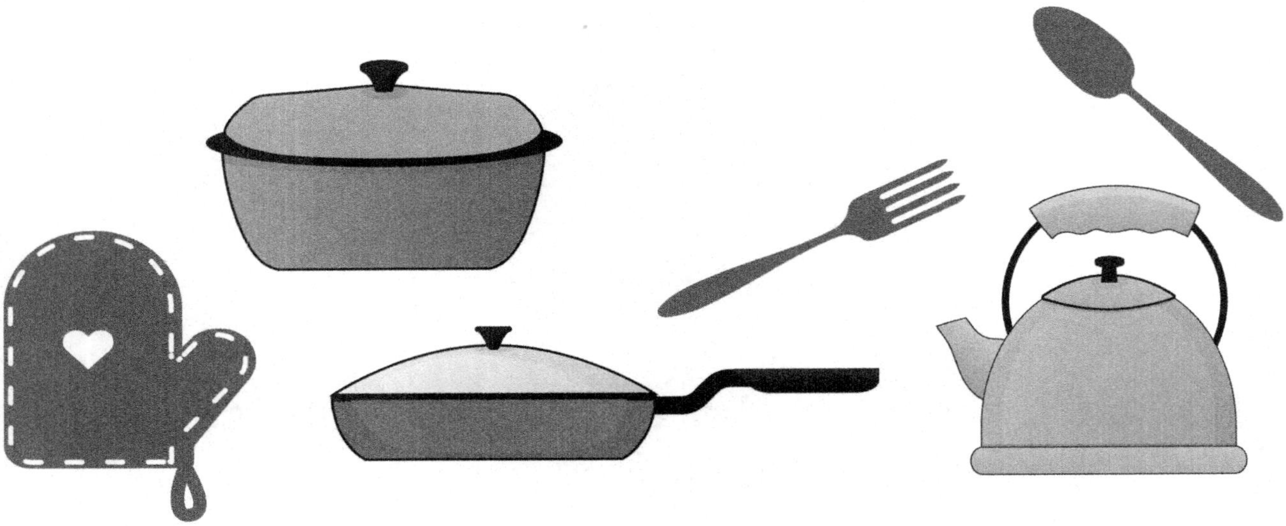

Picture Two

Circle the item you memorized.

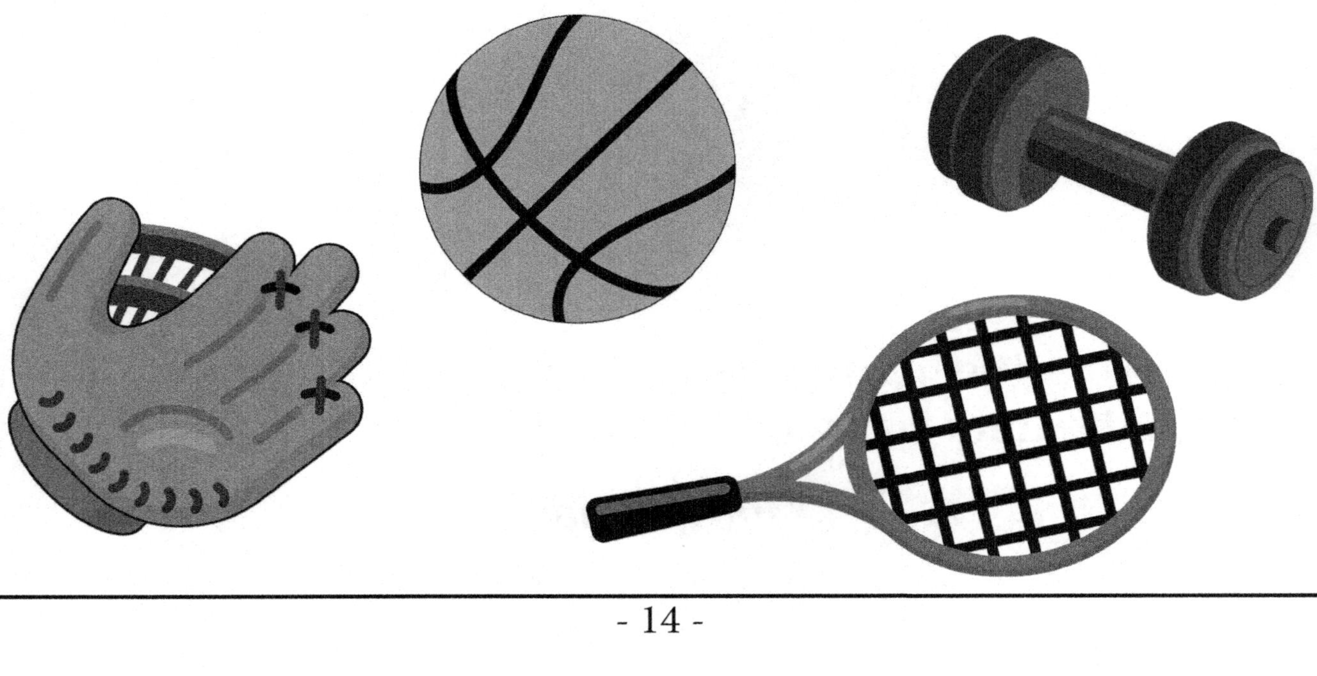

Find the Picture

Picture One:

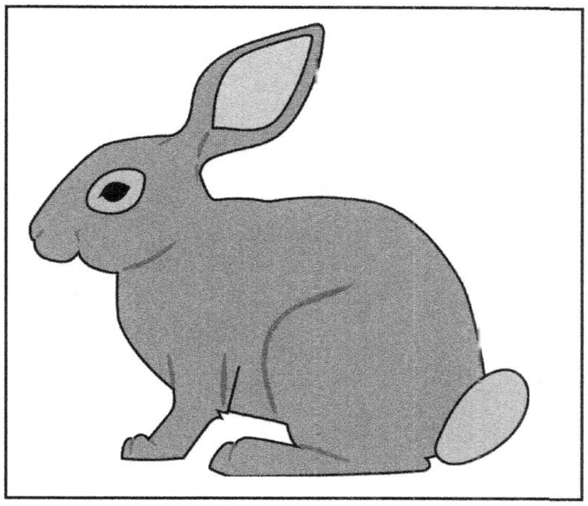

Memorize the item above. Then turn the page, and circle the item you memorized.

turn the page

Picture Two:

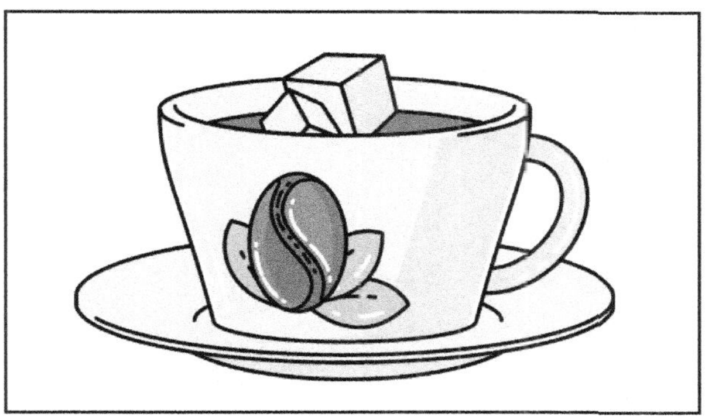

Memorize the item above. Then turn the page, and circle the item you memorized.

turn the page

Puzzle continued from the previous page.

Picture One

Circle the item you memorized.

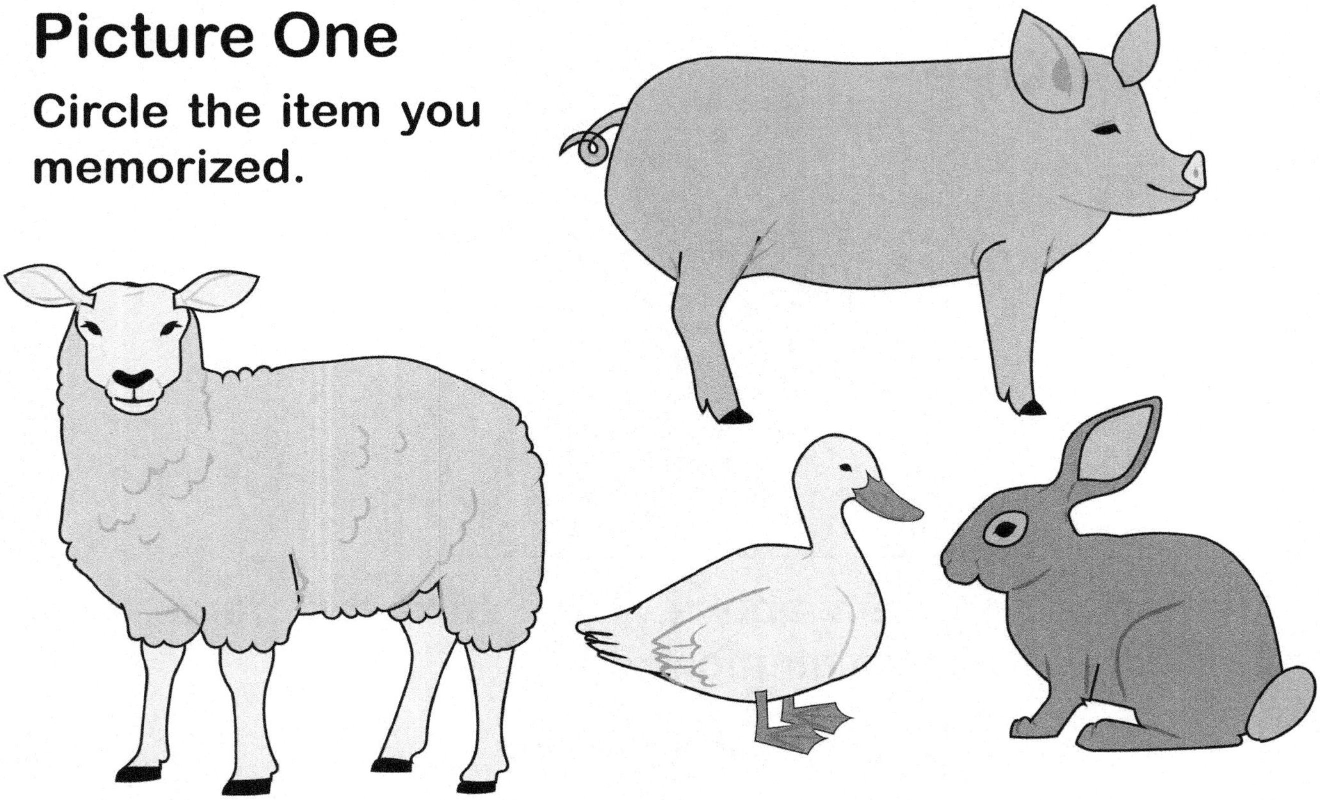

Picture Two

Circle the item you memorized.

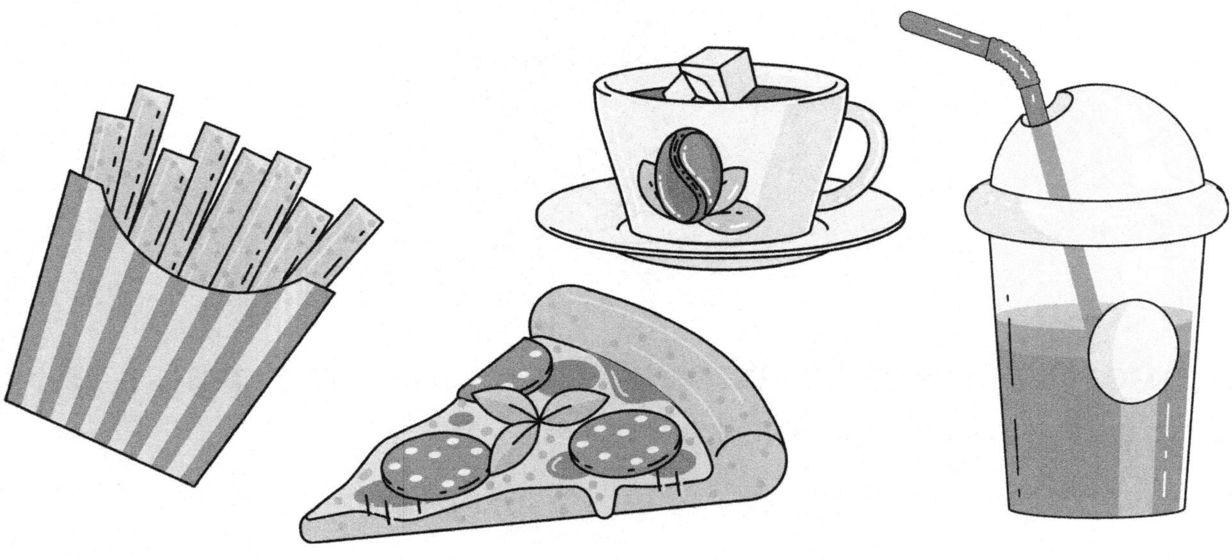

Find the Picture

Picture One:

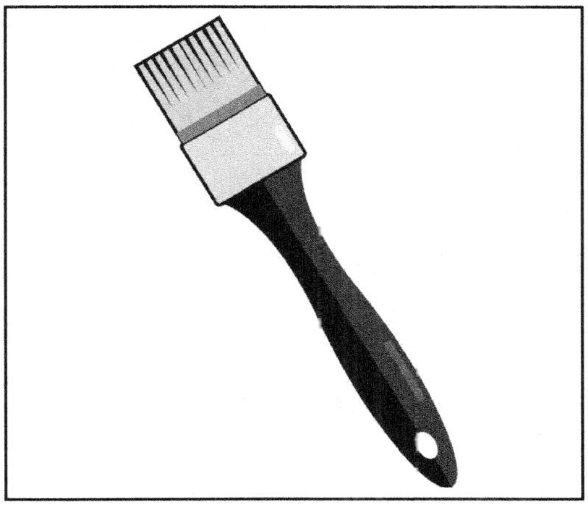

Memorize the item above. Then turn the page, and circle the item you memorized.

turn the page

Picture Two:

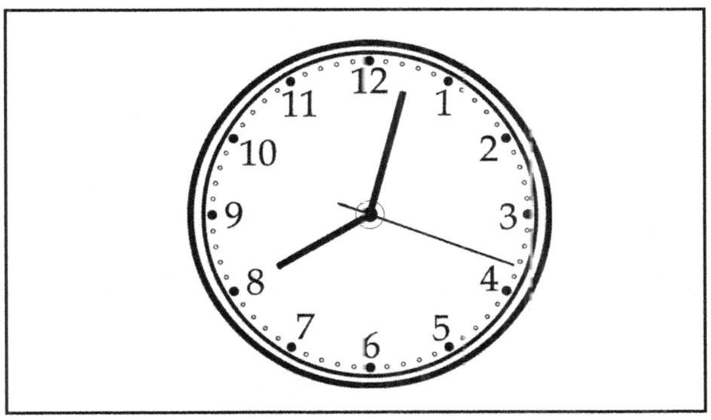

Memorize the item above. Then turn the page, and circle the item you memorized.

turn the page

Memory Game

Puzzle continued from the previous page.

Picture One

Circle the item you memorized.

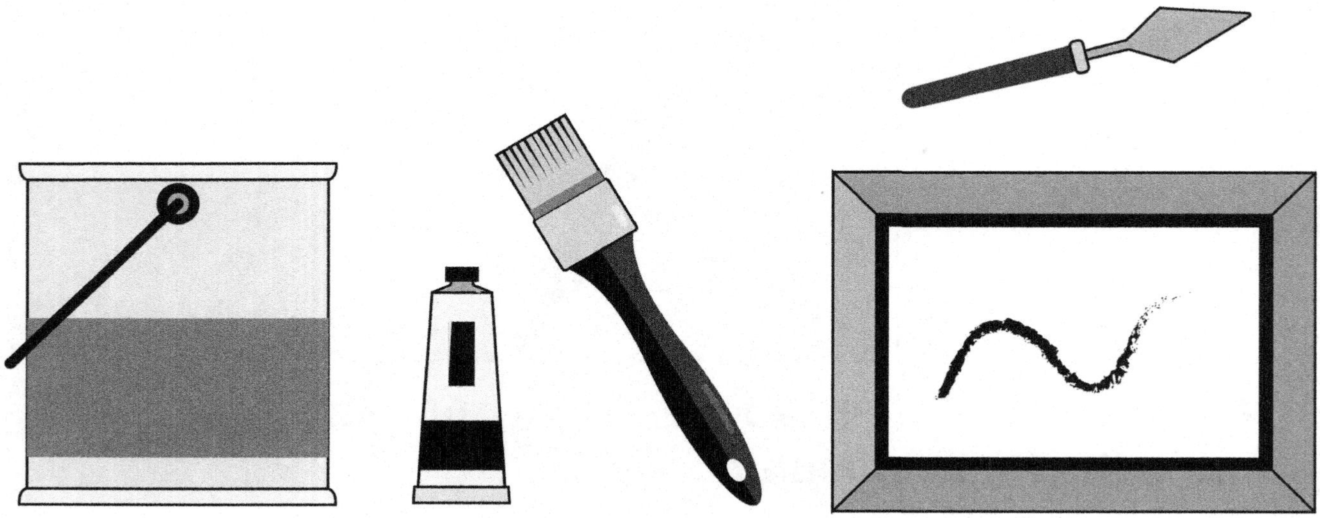

Picture Two

Circle the item you memorized.

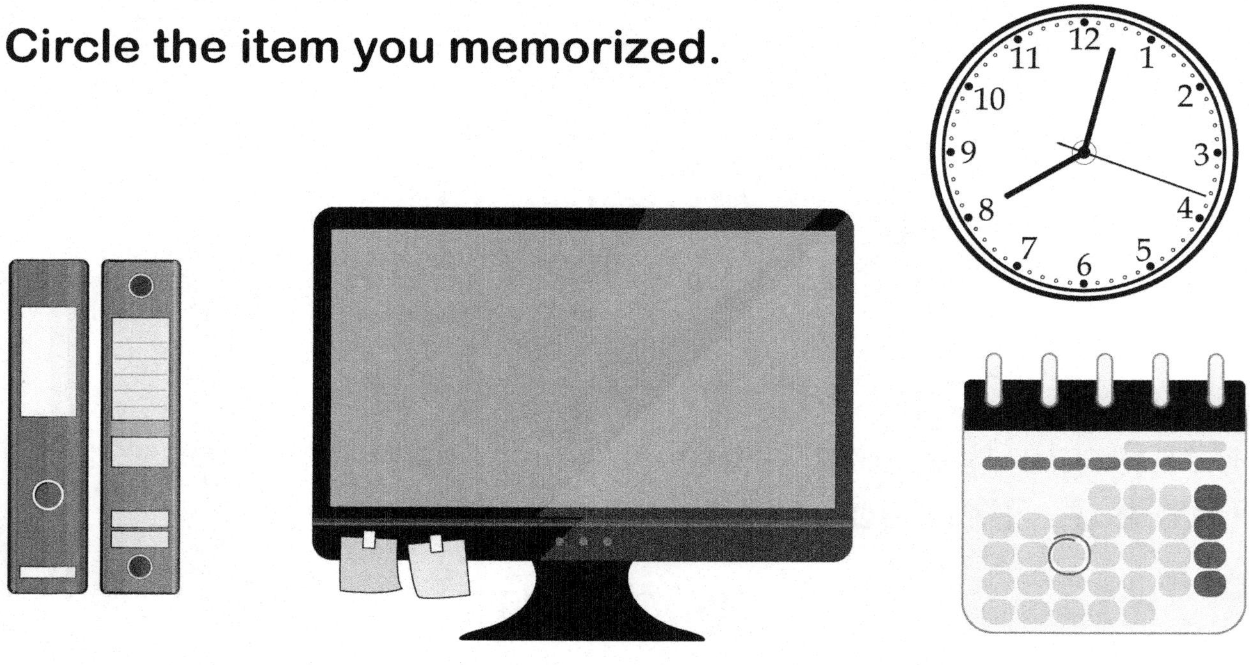

Section Two
Fun Puzzles

SPOT THE ODD ONE OUT

HOW TO PLAY

Spot the Odd One Out

1. Take a look at the pictures.

2. Find and circle the one picture that is different from the rest.

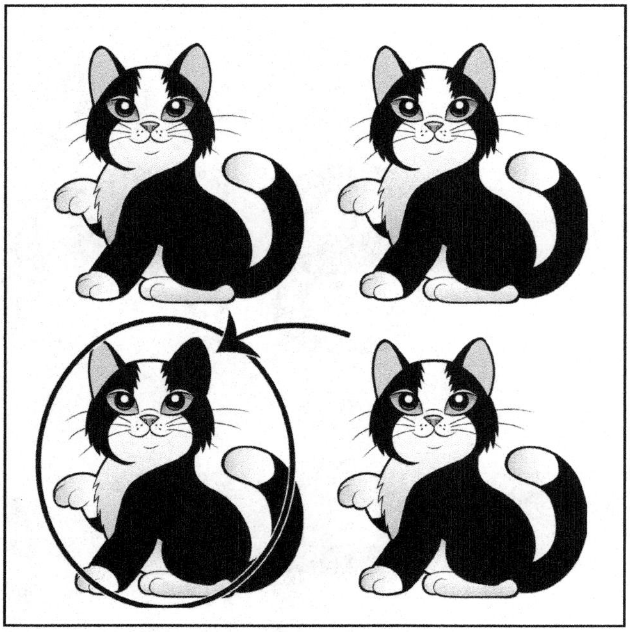

Helpful Hints!

✓ If you are having a hard time finding the picture that is different, try checking each picture in a specific area. In the example above, you need to compare each cat's ear to find the picture that is different.

✓ Take your time looking for the picture that is different. Also, you can always skip a puzzle, and come back to it later.

Fun Puzzle

SPOT THE ODD ONE OUT

FIND THE TEAPOT THAT IS DIFFERENT FROM THE REST

Fun Puzzle

SPOT THE ODD ONE OUT

FIND THE CUPCAKE THAT IS DIFFERENT FROM THE REST

SPOT THE ODD ONE OUT

FIND THE FOX THAT IS DIFFERENT FROM THE REST

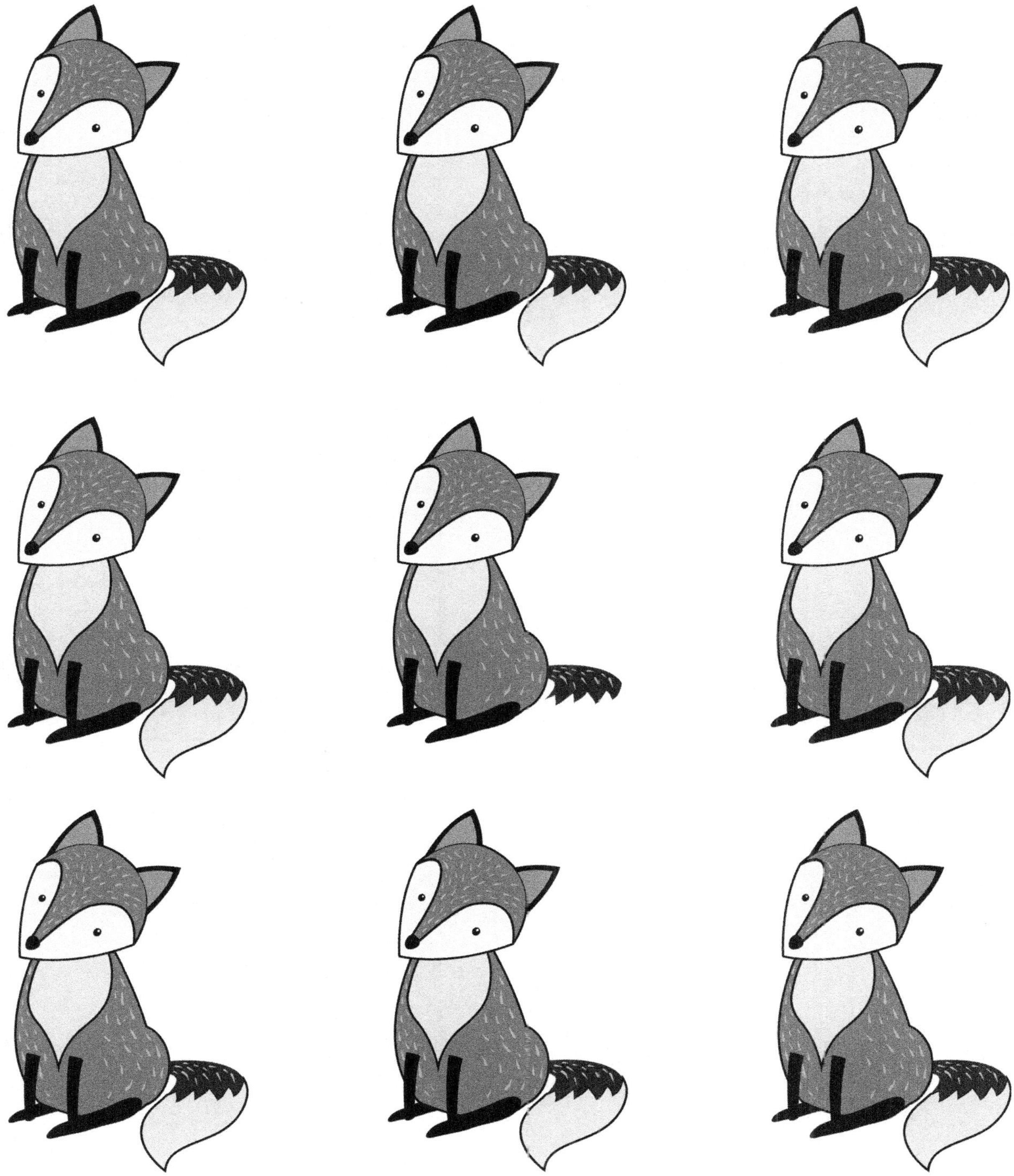

Fun Puzzle

SPOT THE ODD ONE OUT

FIND THE CHAIR THAT IS DIFFERENT FROM THE REST

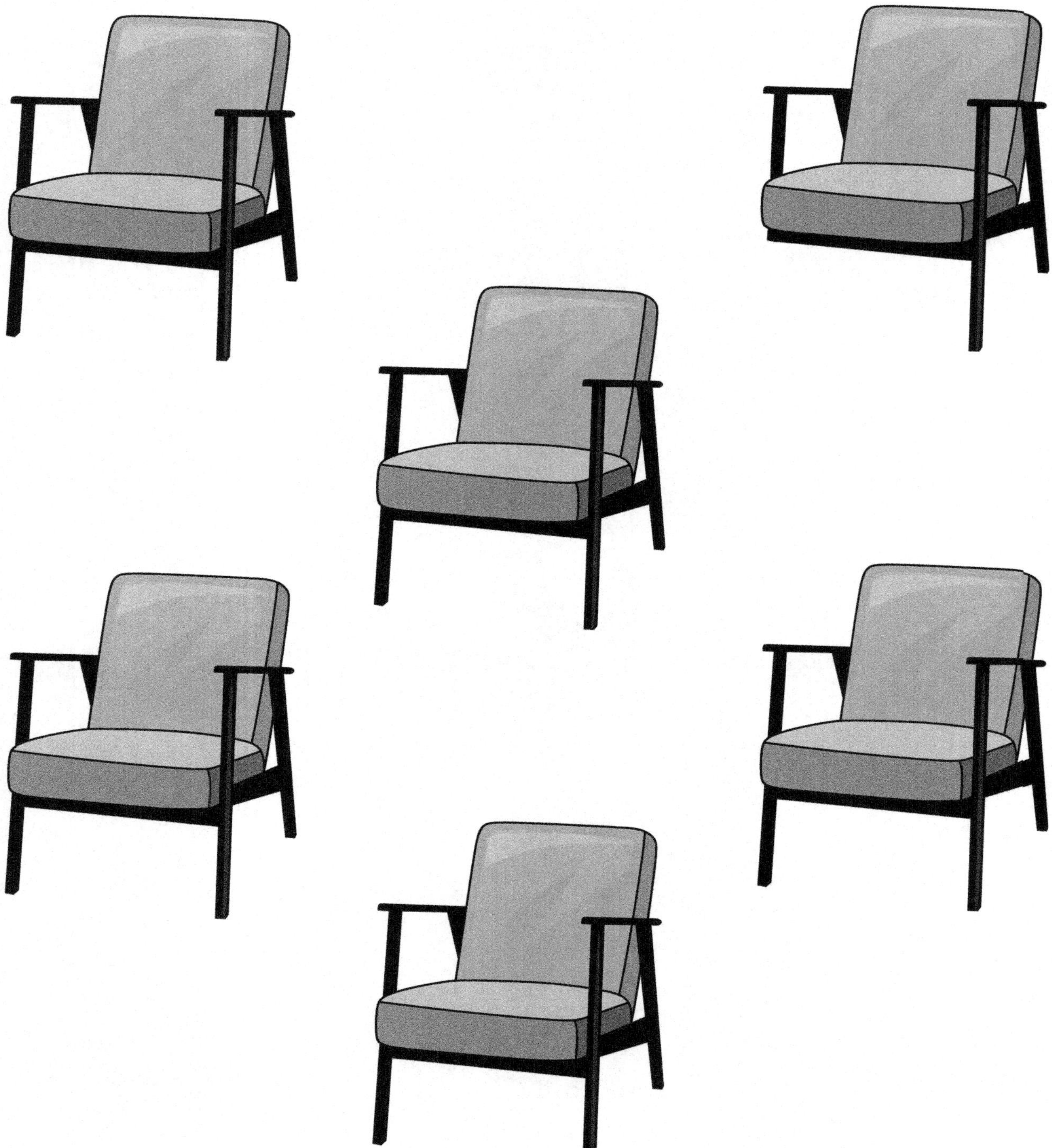

SPOT THE ODD ONE OUT

FIND THE TV THAT IS DIFFERENT FROM THE REST

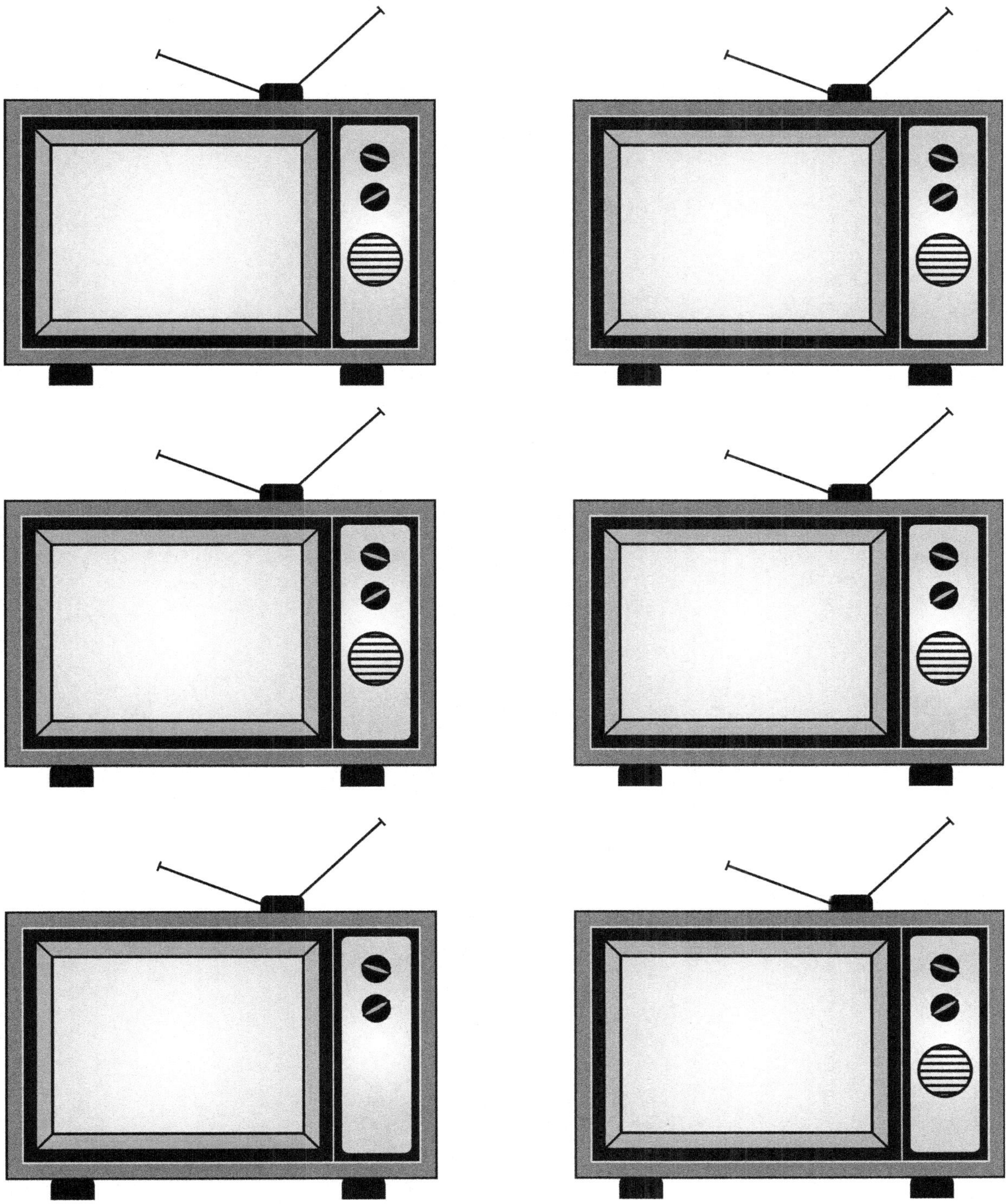

Fun Puzzle

SPOT THE ODD ONE OUT

FIND THE FLOWER THAT IS DIFFERENT FROM THE REST

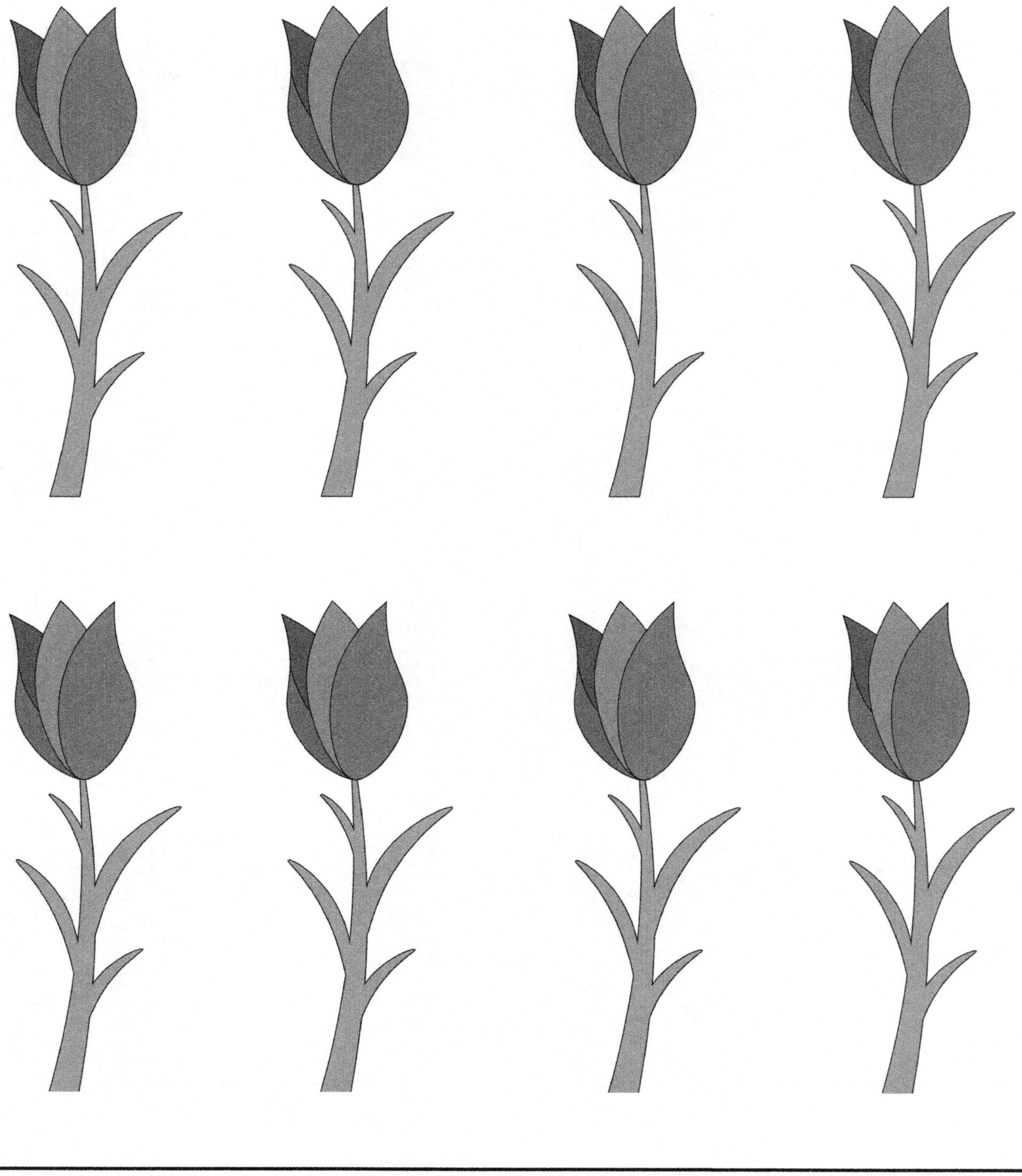

SPOT THE ODD ONE OUT

FIND THE PAIR OF RUBBER BOOTS THAT IS DIFFERENT FROM THE REST

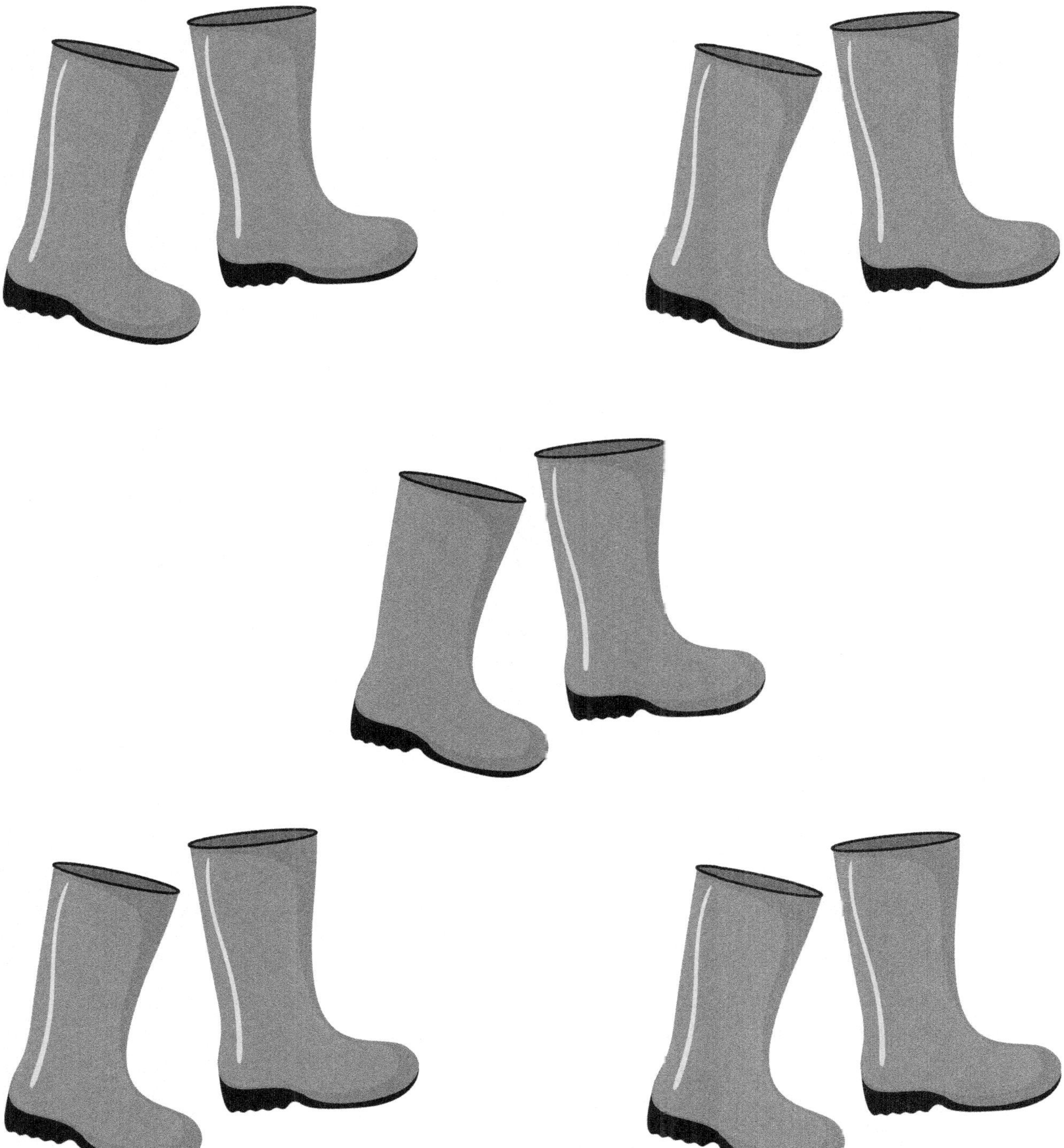

Fun Puzzle

SPOT THE ODD ONE OUT

FIND THE TREE THAT IS DIFFERENT FROM THE REST

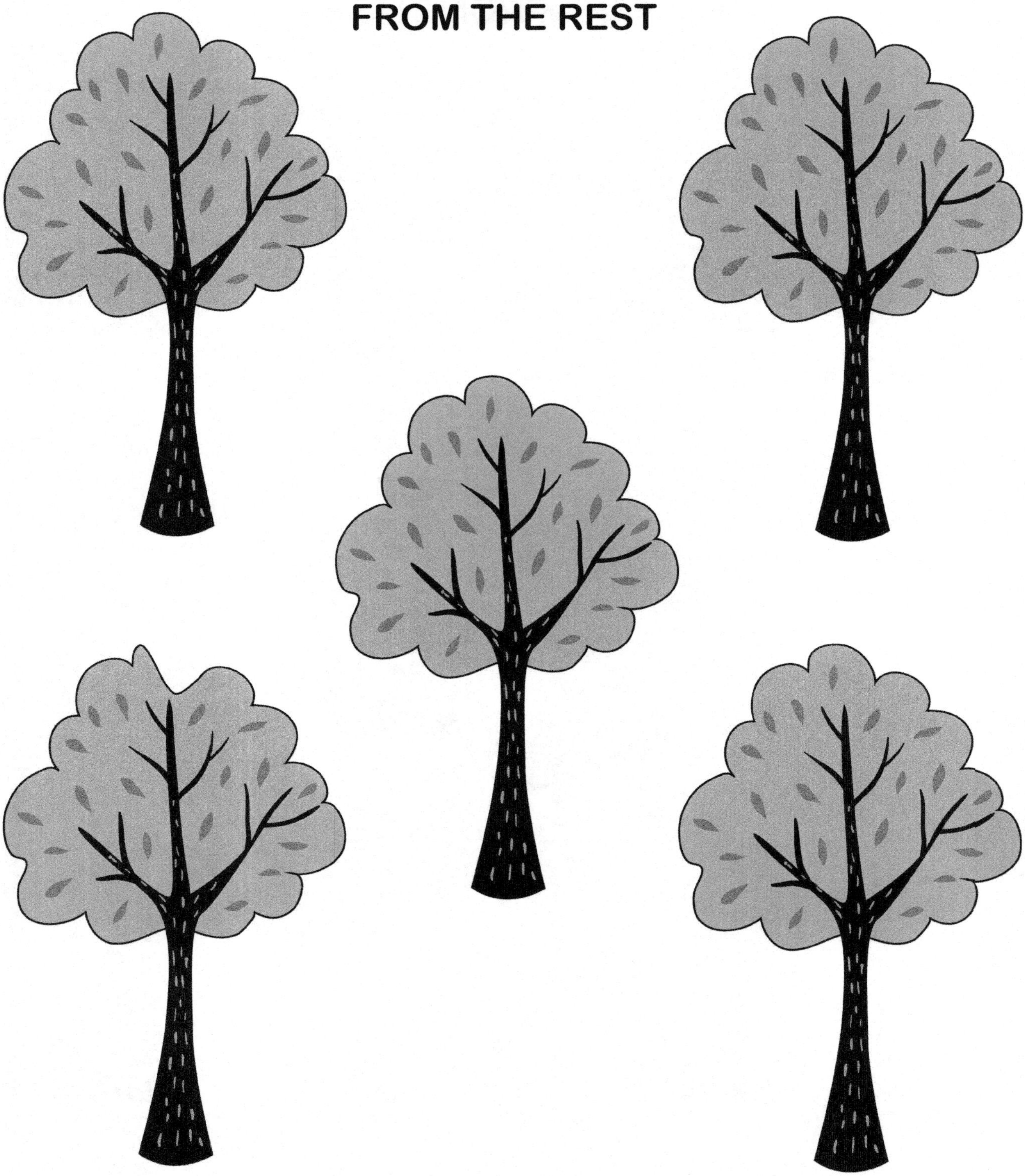

Fun Puzzle

SPOT THE ODD ONE OUT

FIND THE BIRD THAT IS DIFFERENT FROM THE REST

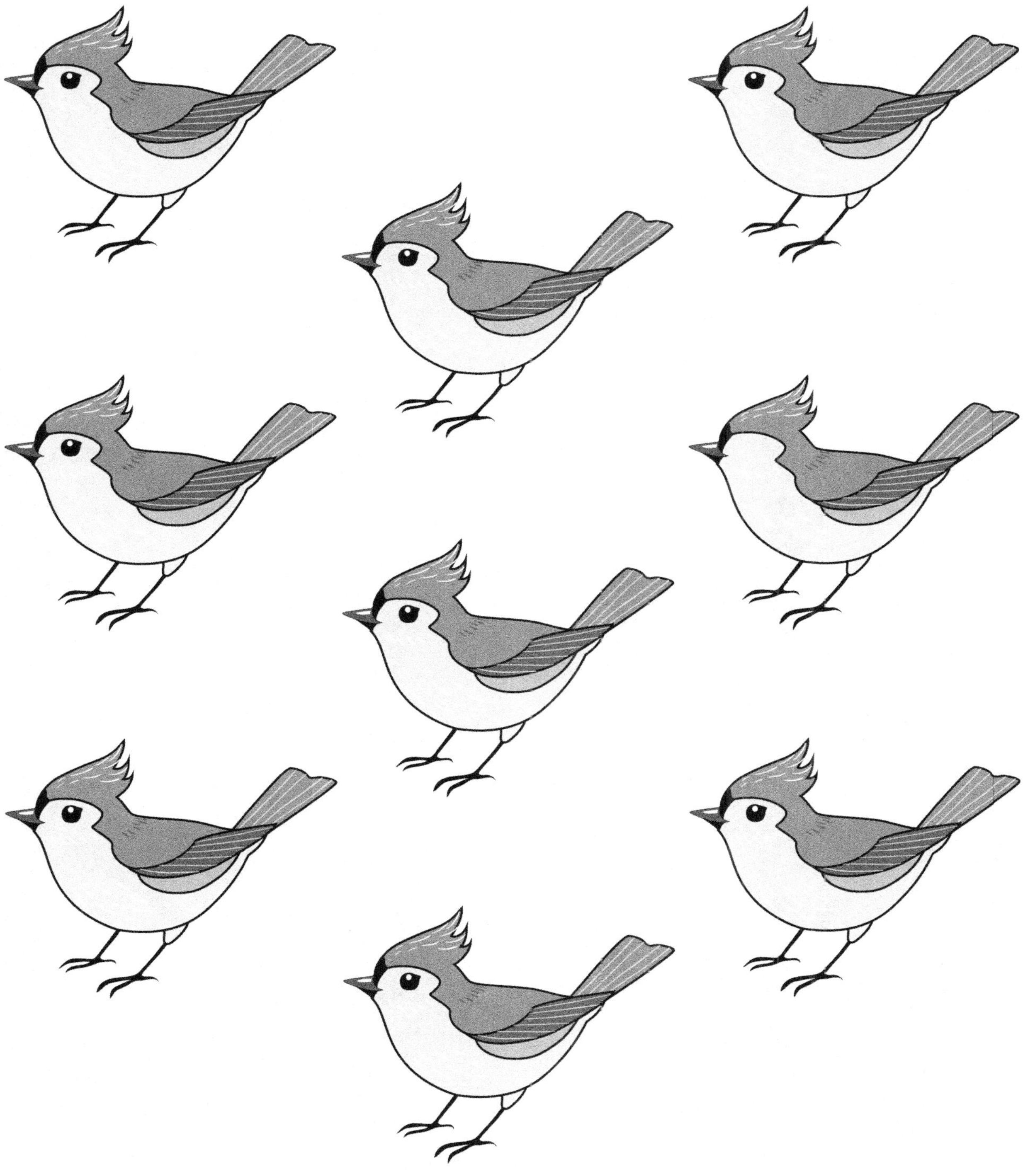

Fun Puzzle

SPOT THE ODD ONE OUT

FIND THE BUTTERFLY THAT IS DIFFERENT FROM THE REST

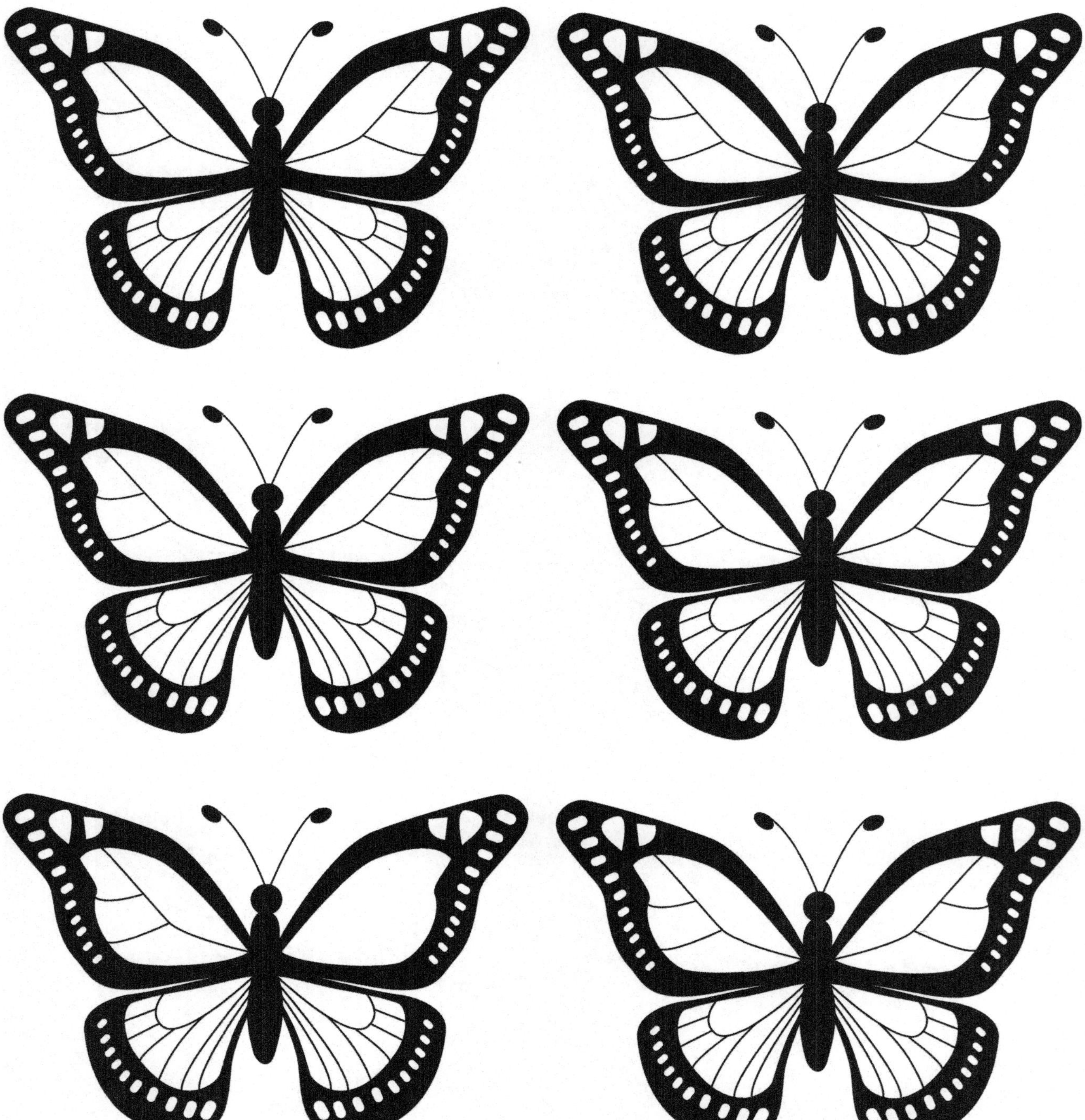

Fun Puzzle

SPOT THE ODD ONE OUT

FIND THE PURSE THAT IS DIFFERENT
FROM THE REST

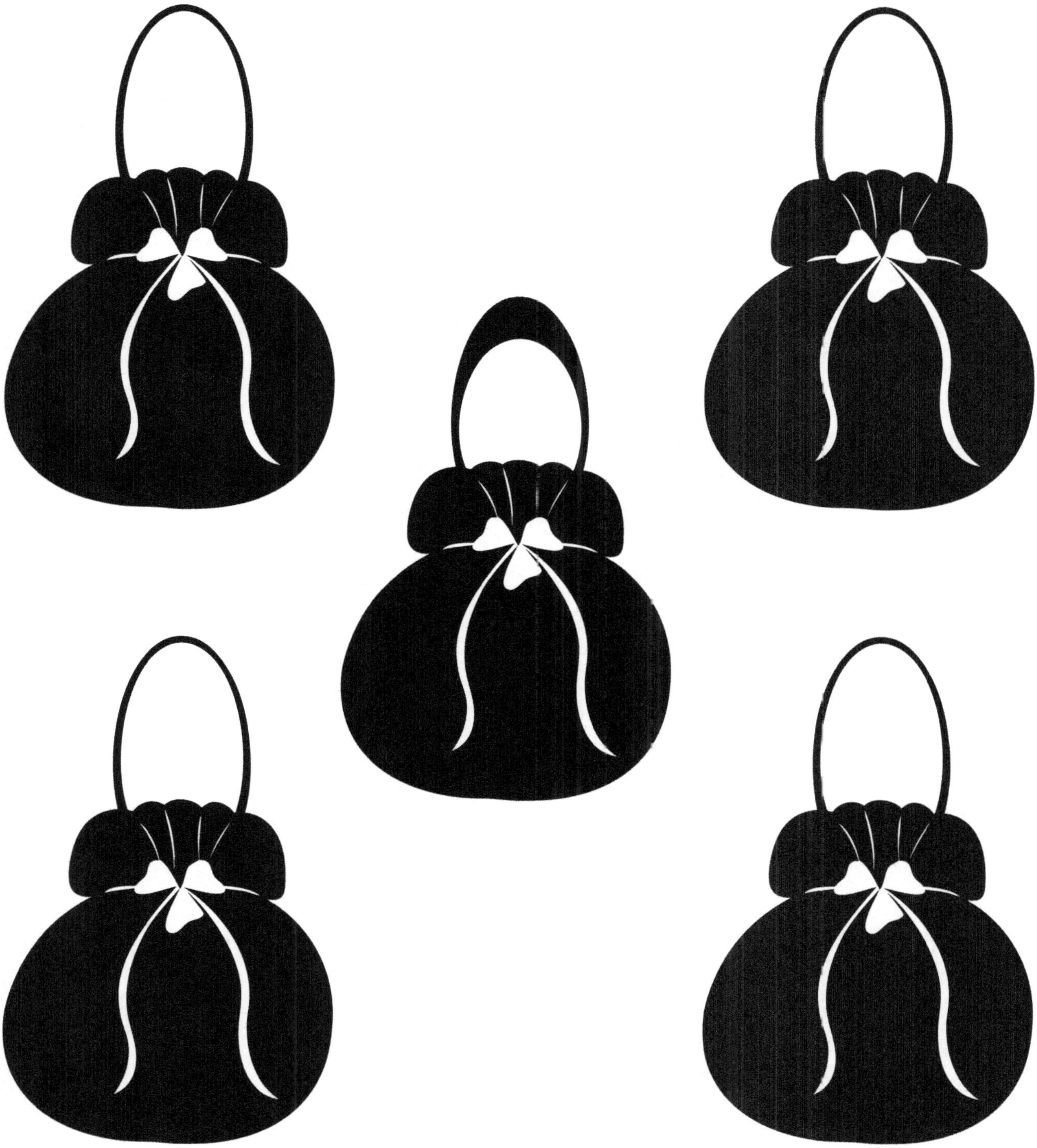

Fun Puzzle

SPOT THE ODD ONE OUT

FIND THE JAR OF HONEY THAT IS DIFFERENT
FROM THE REST

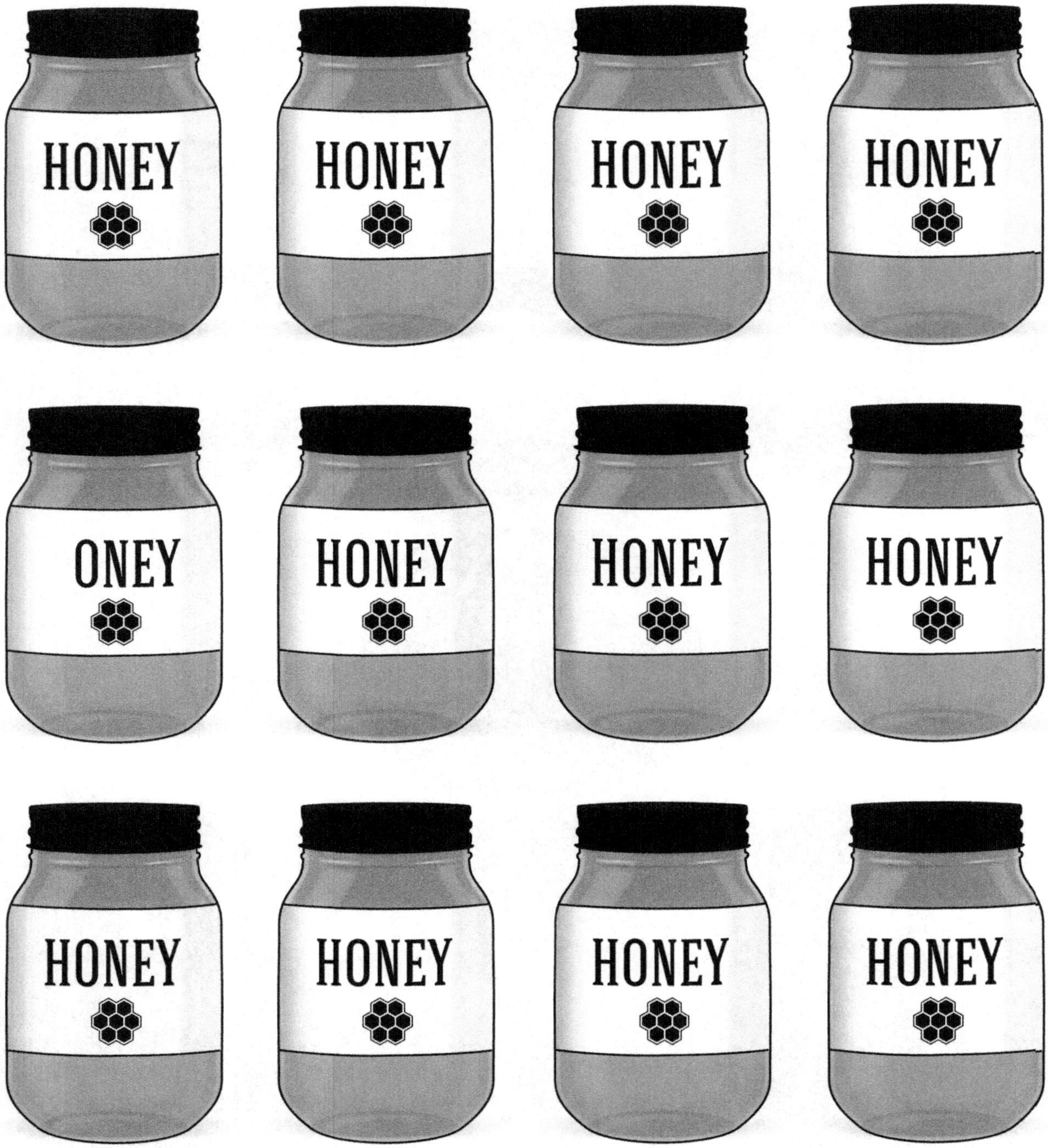

Section Three

Memory Games

FAVORITE NUMBER

HOW TO PLAY

Favorite Number

1. Memorize the favorite number.

   2

2. Turn the page.
3. Circle the number you remember.

   7 3

   (2) 1 5

Helpful Hints!

✓ If you are having a hard time remembering a number, try to relate the number to everyday life. In the example above, you could remember — you have two hands — to help remember the number two.

✓ Take your time memorizing the number. And feel free to try each memory game as many times as you would like.

Favorite Number

Lisa's favorite number is:

7

Memorize the number above. Then turn the page, and pick out the number from a selection of numbers.

turn the page

Edward's favorite number is:

9

Memorize the number above. Then turn the page, and pick out the number from a selection of numbers.

turn the page

Memory Game

Puzzle continued from the previous page.

Which number is Lisa's favorite?

Circle the number that you remember from the previous page.

2 3 5 7 9

Which number is Edward's favorite?

Circle the number that you remember from the previous page.

4 9 1 0 2

Favorite Number

John's favorite number is:

8

Memorize the number above. Then turn the page, and pick out the number from a selection of numbers.

turn the page

Elaine's favorite number is:

3

Memorize the number above. Then turn the page, and pick out the number from a selection of numbers.

turn the page

Memory Game

Puzzle continued from the previous page.

Which number is John's favorite?

Circle the number that you remember from the previous page.

1 0 9

8 6

Which number is Elaine's favorite?

Circle the number that you remember from the previous page.

2 1 3

7 4

Favorite Number

Rachel's favorite number is:

4

Memorize the number above. Then turn the page, and pick out the number from a selection of numbers.

turn the page

William's favorite number is:

0

Memorize the number above. Then turn the page, and pick out the number from a selection of numbers.

turn the page

Puzzle continued from the previous page.

Which number is Rachel's favorite?

Circle the number that you remember from the previous page.

7 2 4 3 6

Which number is William's favorite?

Circle the number that you remember from the previous page.

9 0 5 2 1

Favorite Number

Preston's favorite number is:

23

Memorize the number above. Then turn the page, and pick out the number from a selection of numbers.

turn the page

Larry's favorite number is:

15

Memorize the number above. Then turn the page, and pick out the number from a selection of numbers.

turn the page

Memory Game

Puzzle continued from the previous page.

Which number is Preston's favorite?

Circle the number that you remember from the previous page.

23 46

12 30

Which number is Larry's favorite?

Circle the number that you remember from the previous page.

40 28

32 15

Favorite Number

Monica's favorite number is:

14

Memorize the number above. Then turn the page, and pick out the number from a selection of numbers.

turn the page

Frasier's favorite number is:

30

Memorize the number above. Then turn the page, and pick out the number from a selection of numbers.

turn the page

Memory Game

Puzzle continued from the previous page.

Which number is Monica's favorite?

Circle the number that you remember from the previous page.

32 14

21 53

Which number is Frasier's favorite?

Circle the number that you remember from the previous page.

15 26

30 18

Favorite Number

Jamie's favorite number is:

25

Memorize the number above. Then turn the page, and pick out the number from a selection of numbers.

turn the page

Kate's favorite number is:

11

Memorize the number above. Then turn the page, and pick out the number from a selection of numbers.

turn the page

Puzzle continued from the previous page.

Which number is Jamie's favorite?

Circle the number that you remember from the previous page.

51 17

42 25

Which number is Kate's favorite?

Circle the number that you remember from the previous page.

37 62

11 29

Section Four

Fun Puzzles

FIND THE DIFFERENCES

HOW TO PLAY

FIND 3 DIFFERENCES

1. Take a look at the two pictures on the page.
2. Find and circle 3 differences between the two almost identical pictures.

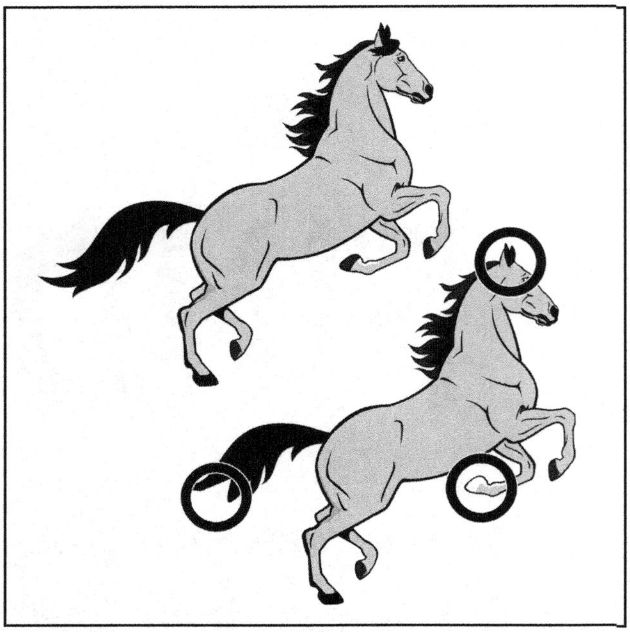

Helpful Hints!

✓ If you are having difficulty finding three differences try comparing the pictures — one specific area at a time. In the example above, you can compare each horse's tail to find a difference.

✓ Take your time looking for the 3 differences. Also, if you get stuck, you can always skip a puzzle, and come back to it later.

FIND 3 DIFFERENCES

FIND THE THREE DIFFERENCES BETWEEN THE TWO PICTURES

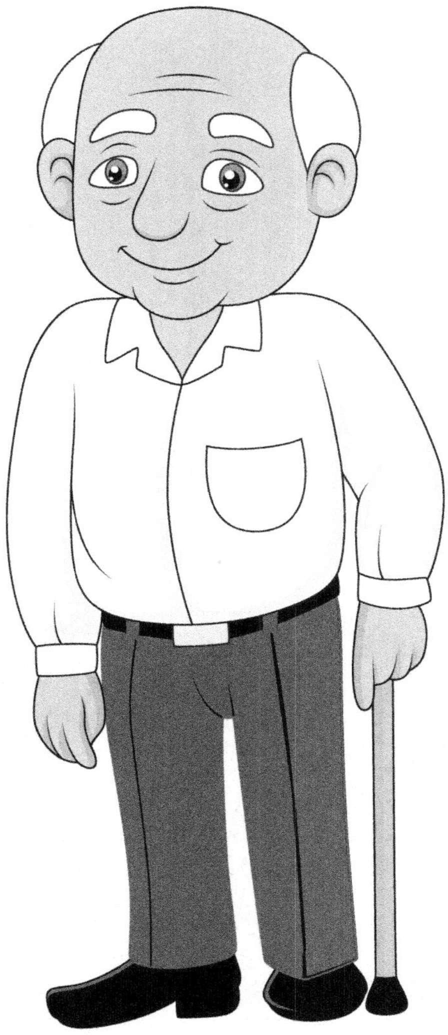

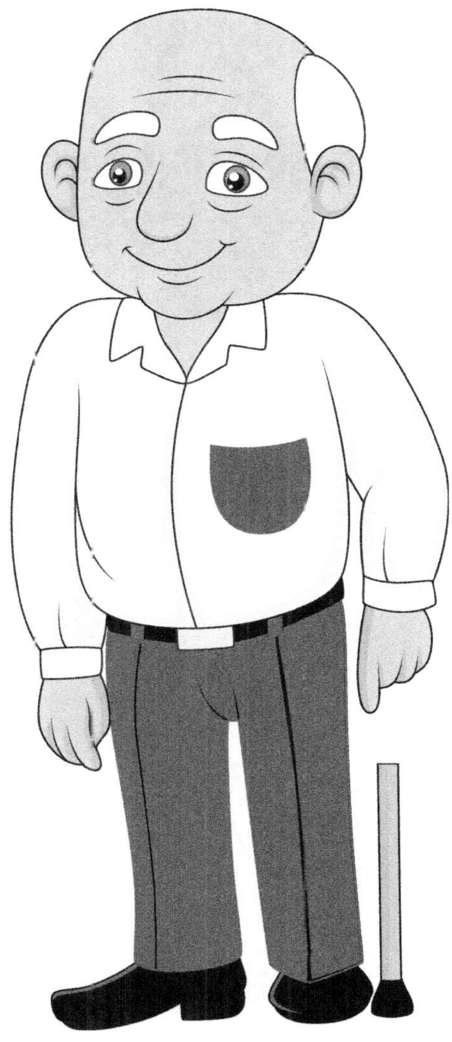

Fun Puzzle

FIND 3 DIFFERENCES

FIND THE THREE DIFFERENCES BETWEEN THE TWO PICTURES

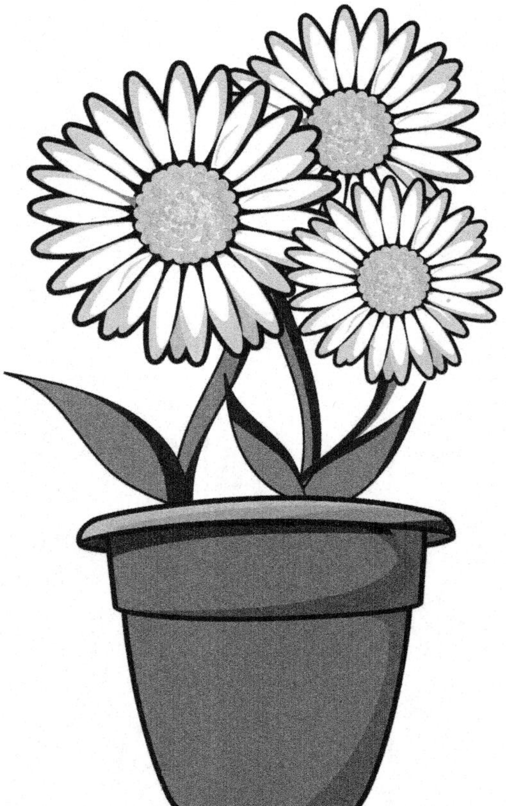

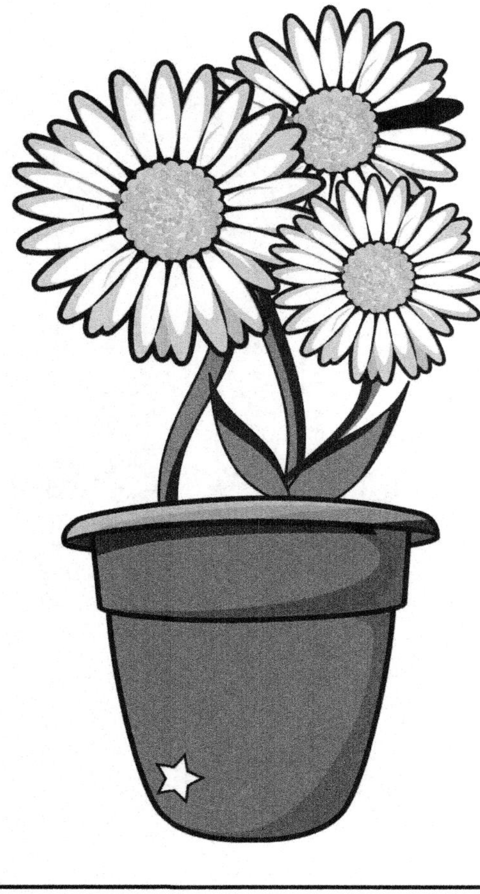

FIND 3 DIFFERENCES

FIND THE THREE DIFFERENCES BETWEEN THE TWO PICTURES

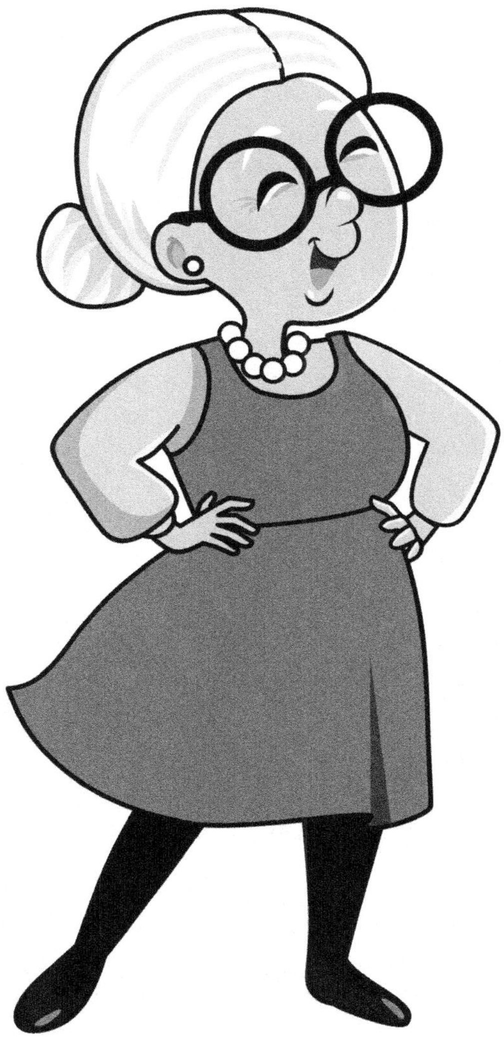

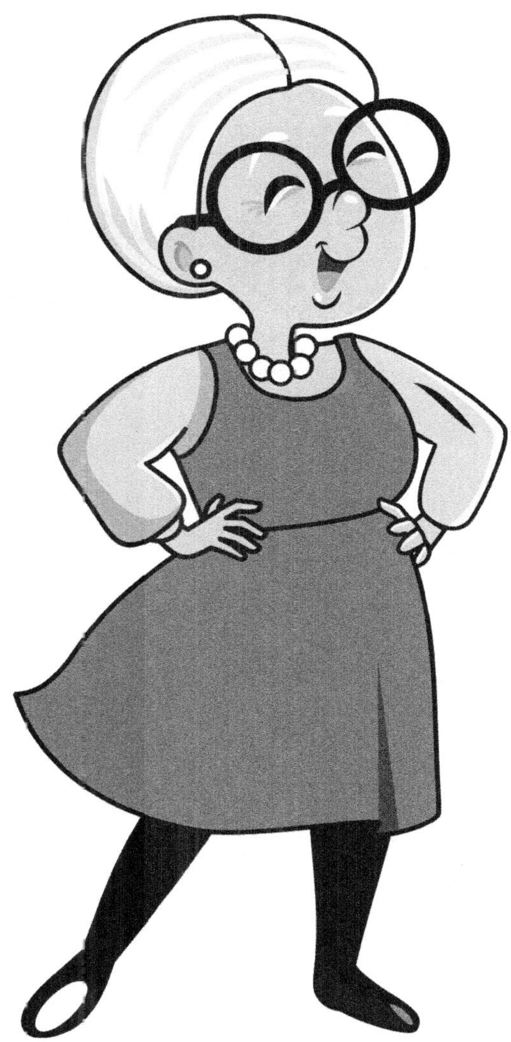

Fun Puzzle

FIND 3 DIFFERENCES

FIND THE THREE DIFFERENCES BETWEEN THE TWO PICTURES

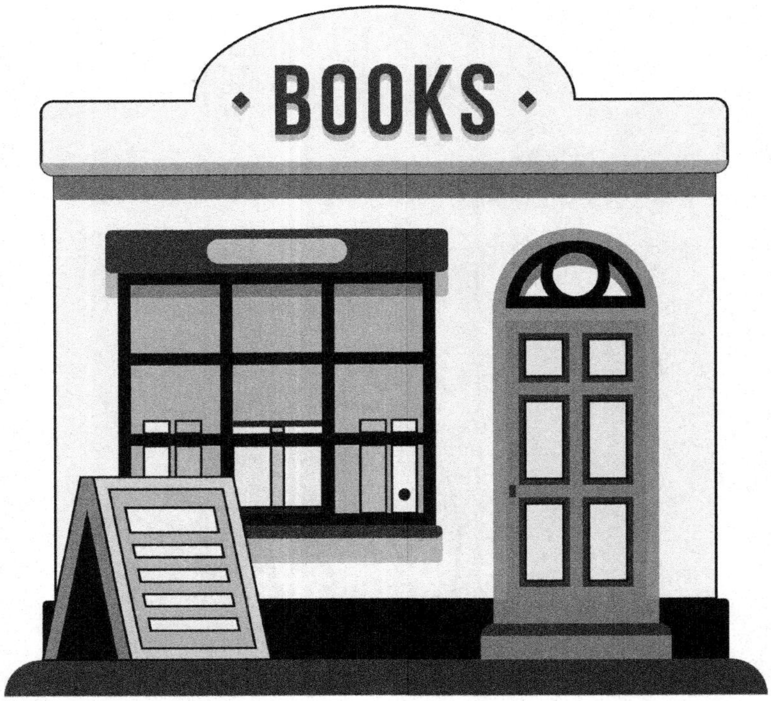

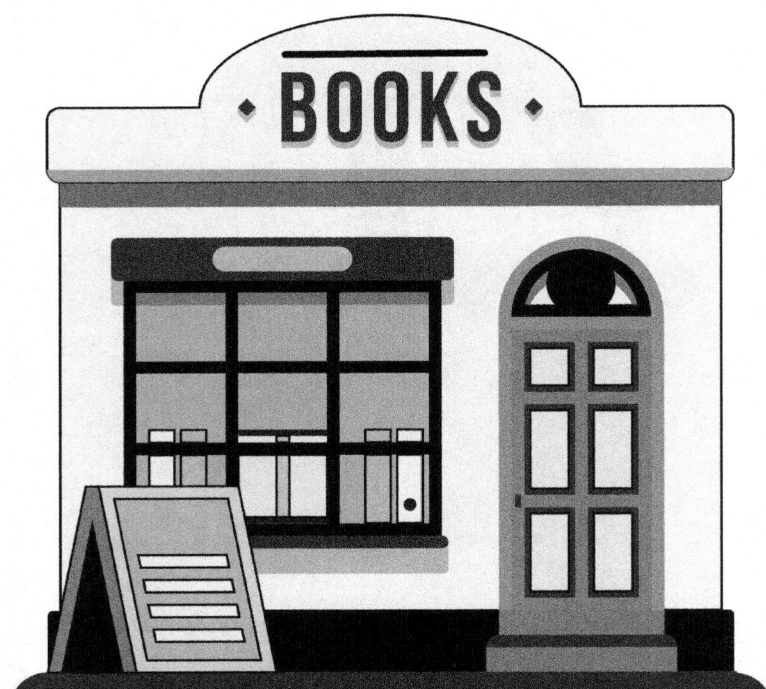

FIND 3 DIFFERENCES

FIND THE THREE DIFFERENCES BETWEEN THE TWO PICTURES

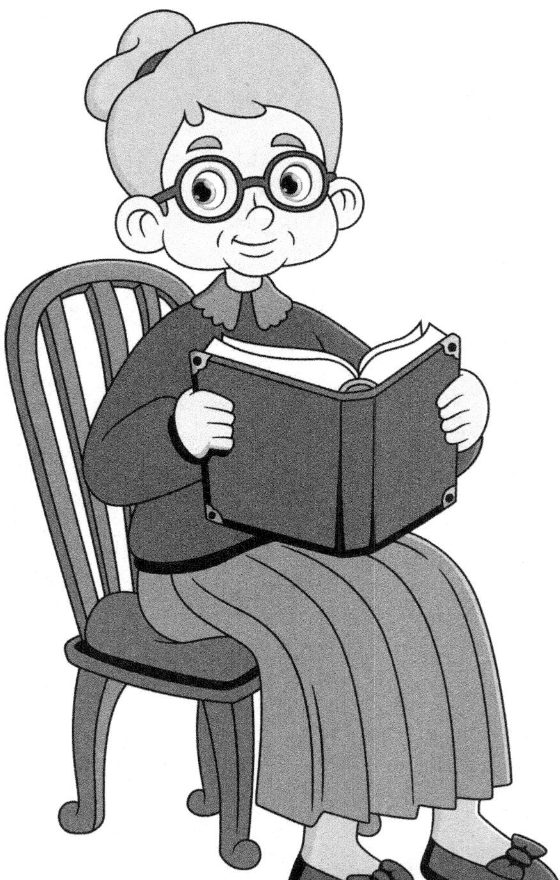

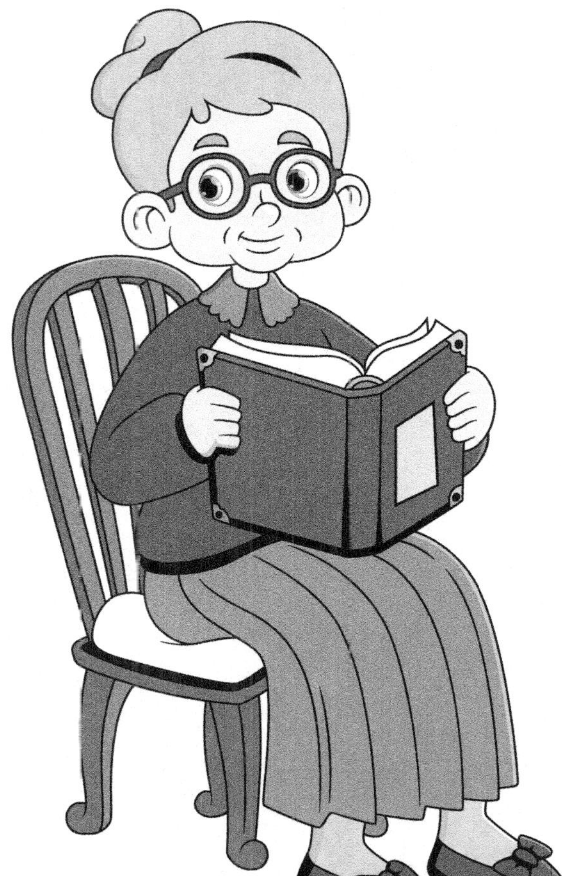

Fun Puzzle

FIND 3 DIFFERENCES

FIND THE THREE DIFFERENCES BETWEEN THE TWO PICTURES

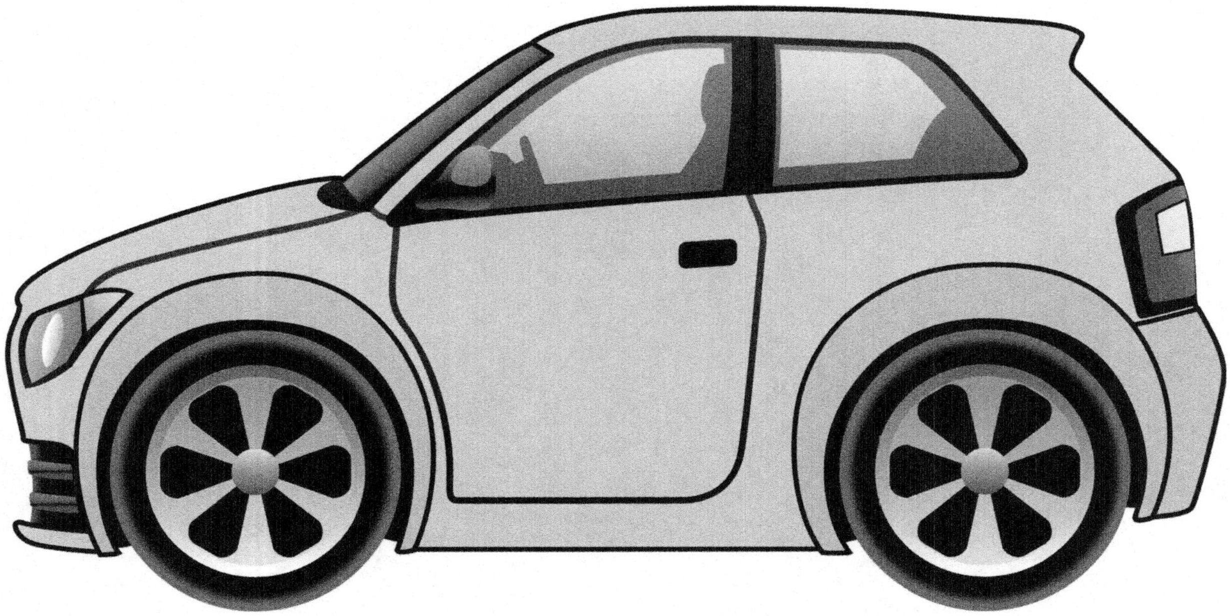

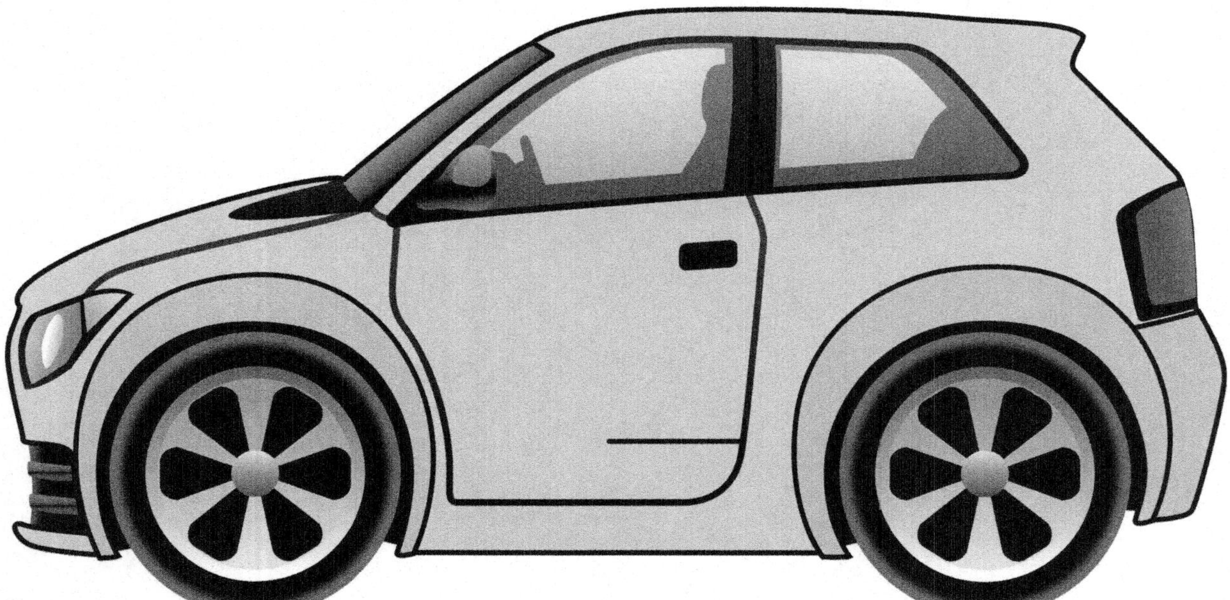

FIND 3 DIFFERENCES

FIND THE THREE DIFFERENCES BETWEEN THE TWO PICTURES

Fun Puzzle

FIND 3 DIFFERENCES

FIND THE THREE DIFFERENCES BETWEEN THE TWO PICTURES

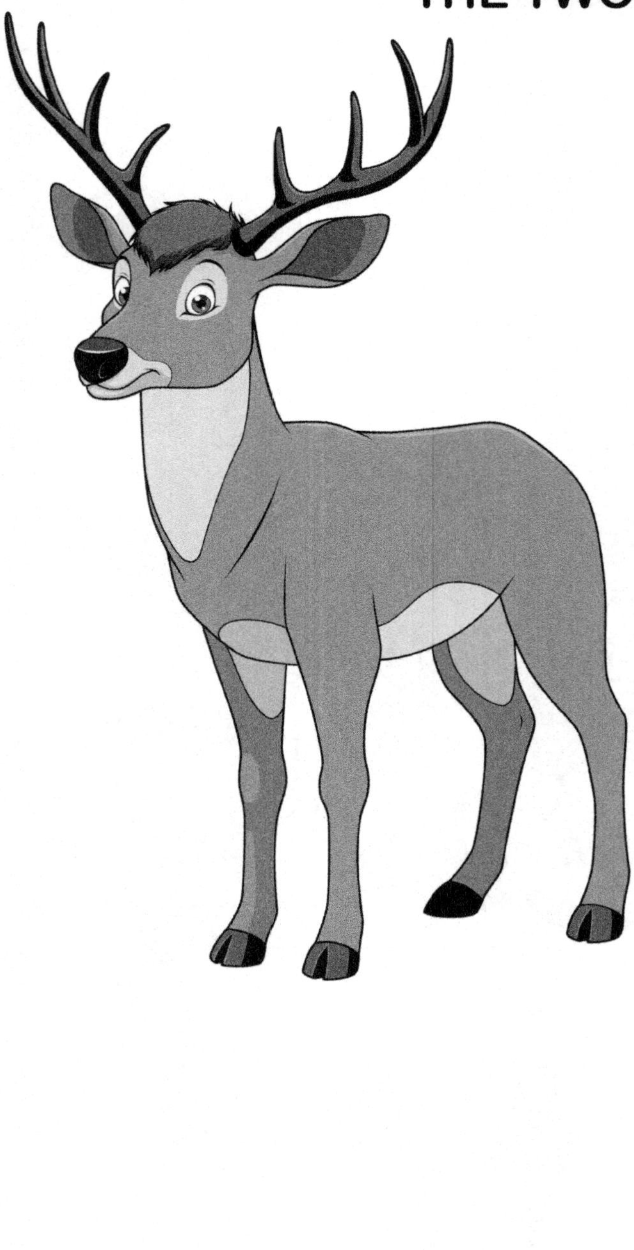

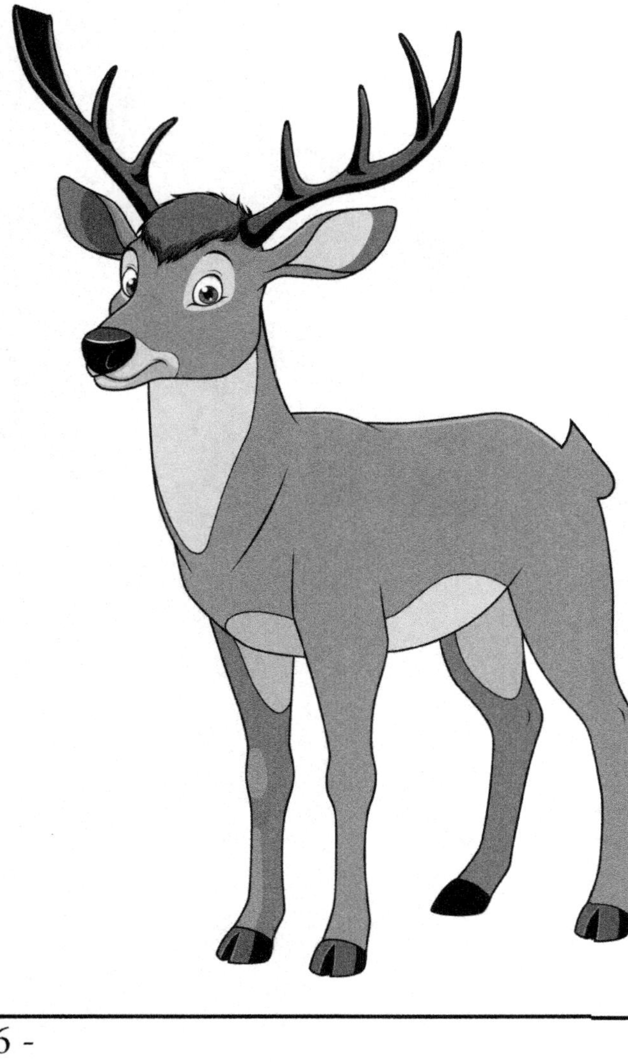

FIND 3 DIFFERENCES

FIND THE THREE DIFFERENCES BETWEEN THE TWO PICTURES

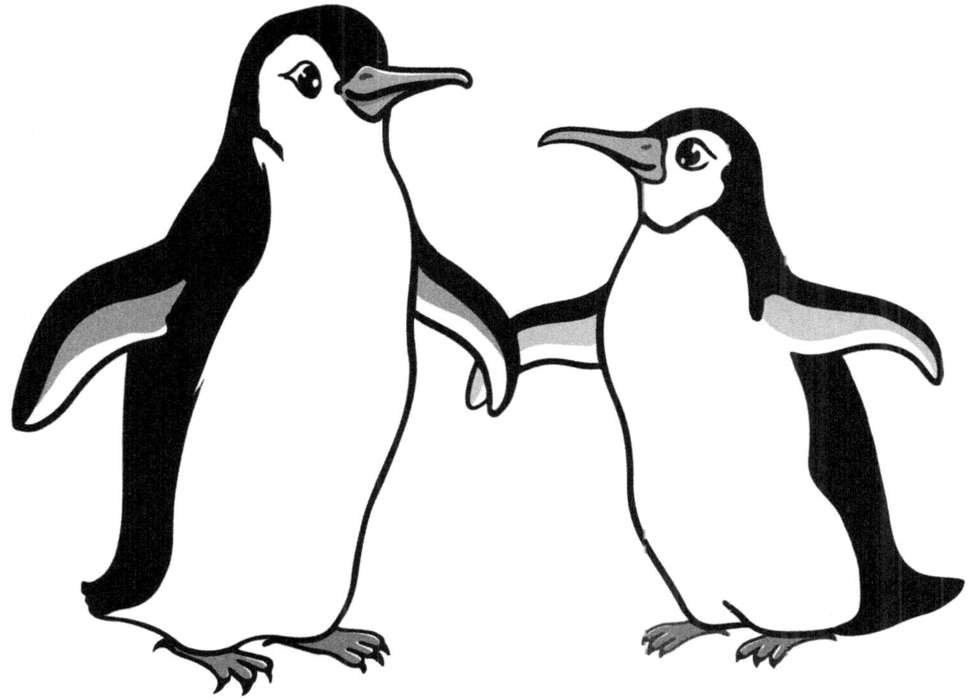

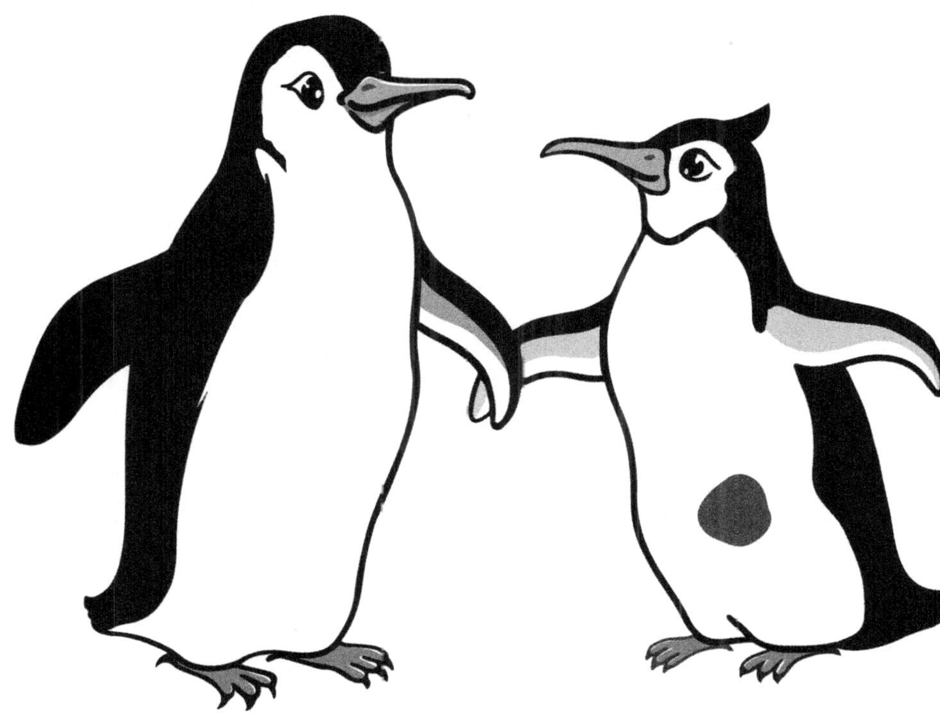

Fun Puzzle

FIND 3 DIFFERENCES

FIND THE THREE DIFFERENCES BETWEEN THE TWO PICTURES

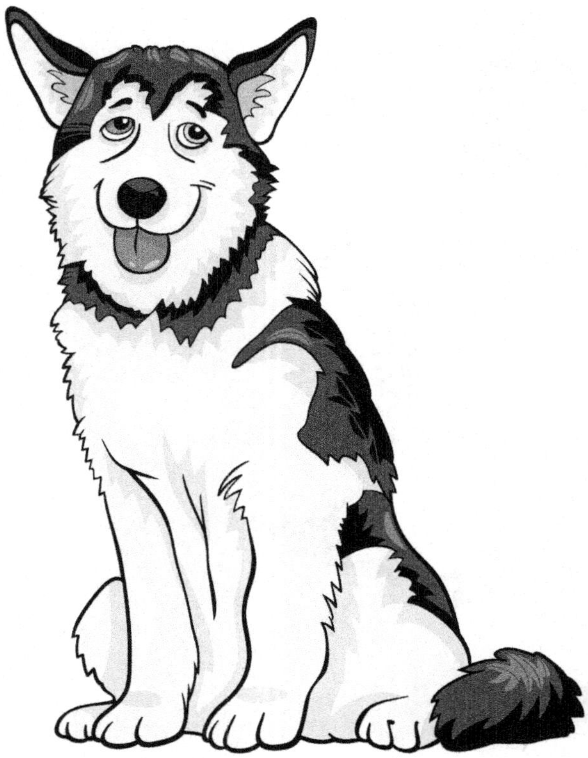

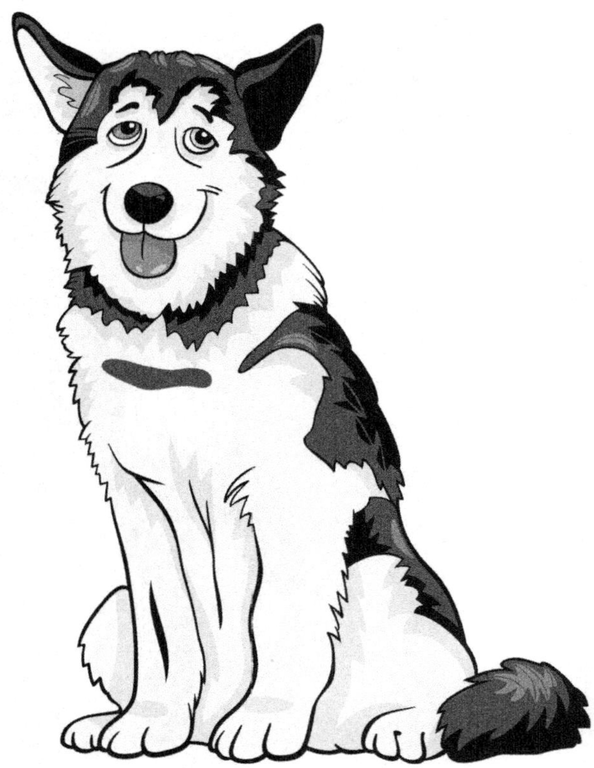

FIND 3 DIFFERENCES

FIND THE THREE DIFFERENCES BETWEEN THE TWO PICTURES

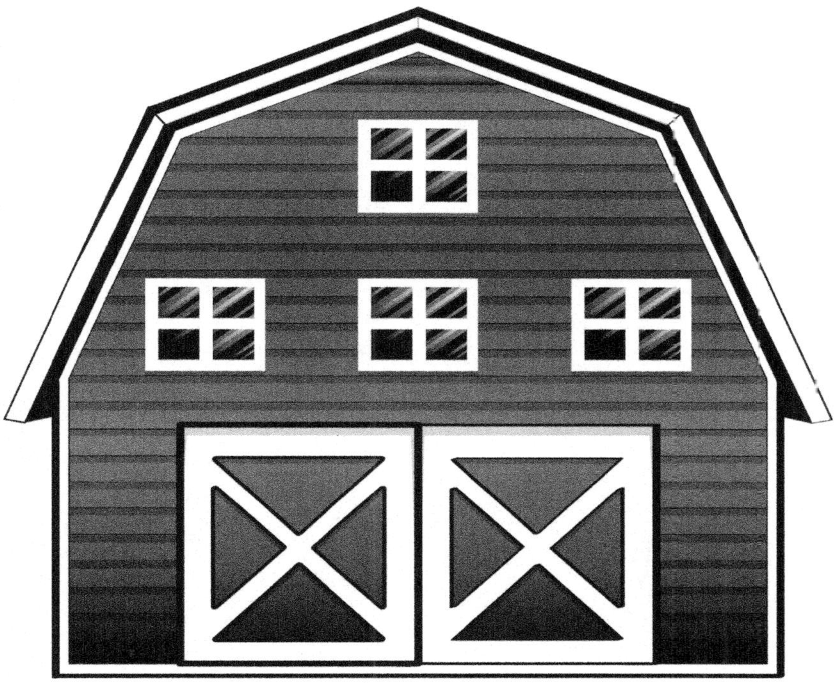

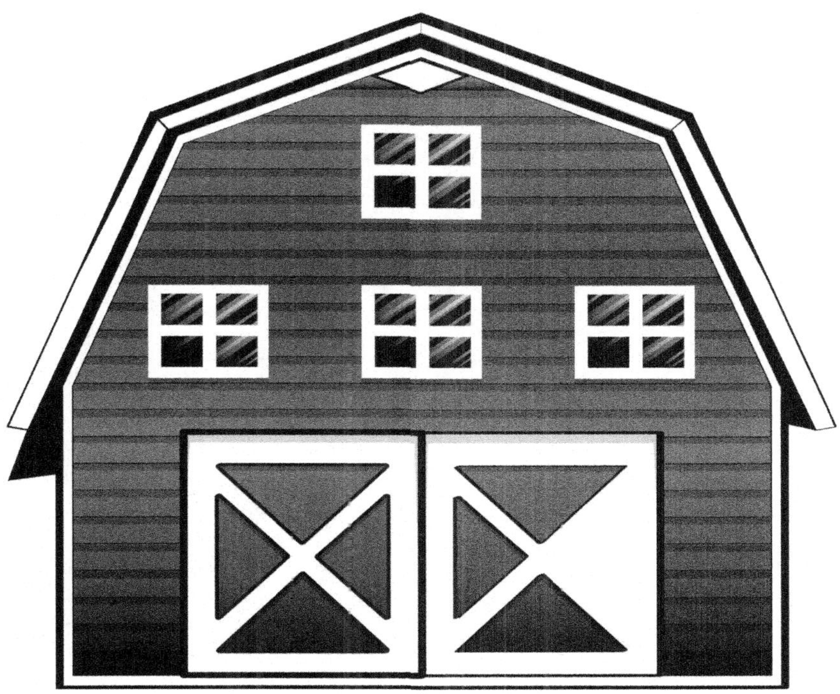

Fun Puzzle

FIND 3 DIFFERENCES

FIND THE THREE DIFFERENCES BETWEEN THE TWO PICTURES

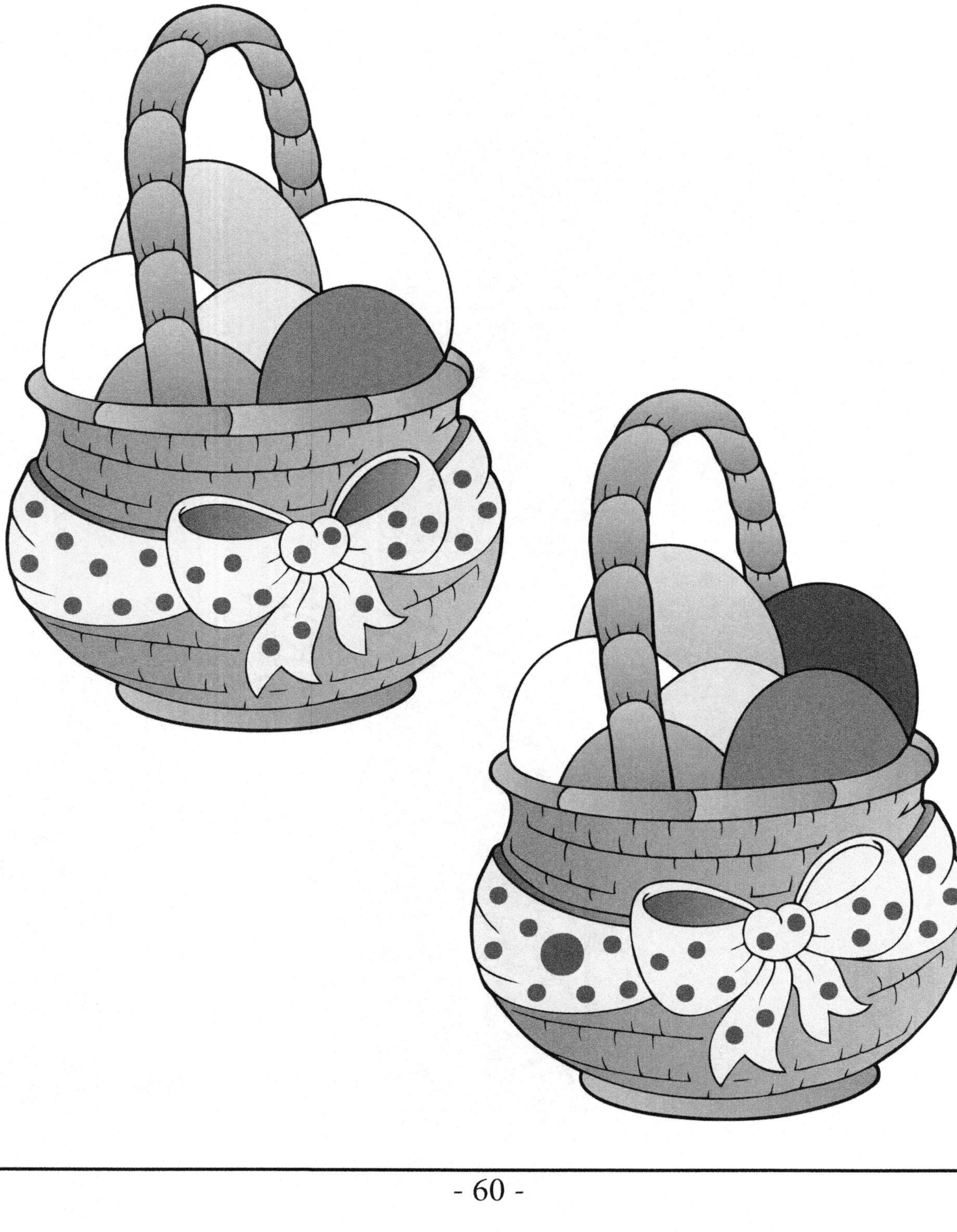

LOVELY WORDS

HOW TO PLAY

Lovely Words

1. Memorize the word located in the box.

candle

2. Turn the page.

3. Circle the word you remember.

tissue	moon
(candle)	salad

Helpful Hints!

✓ To help remember a word, try to relate it to an image of something memorable. In the example above, you could imagine a candle on a birthday cake, to help remember the word 'candle.'

✓ Take your time memorizing the word. And feel free to try each memory game as many times as you would like.

Lovely Words

Word One

Take some time to memorize the word below. Then turn the page and circle the word you remember.

cherry

turn the page

Word Two

Take some time to memorize the word below. Then turn the page and circle the word you remember.

spoon

turn the page

Memory Game

Puzzle continued from the previous page.

Word One

Circle the word you remember from the previous page.

cherry

sun

hamburger

cake

mud

apple

Word Two

Circle the word you remember from the previous page.

fork

plate

hat

cup

spoon

towel

pizza

Lovely Words

Word One

Take some time to memorize the word below. Then turn the page and circle the word you remember.

shirt

turn the page

Word Two

Take some time to memorize the word below. Then turn the page and circle the word you remember.

desk

turn the page

Instructions

Puzzle continued from the previous page.

Word One

Circle the word you remember from the previous page.

shirt glove

sweater dress

pie closet

Word Two

Circle the word you remember from the previous page.

pencil bed

table blanket

chair

book

pillow desk

Lovely Words

Word One

Take some time to memorize the word below. Then turn the page and circle the word you remember.

house

turn the page

Word Two

Take some time to memorize the word below. Then turn the page and circle the word you remember.

tree

turn the page

Memory Game

Puzzle continued from the previous page.

Word One

Circle the word you remember from the previous page.

bird

dog

pool

rabbit

house

stones

forest

Word Two

Circle the word you remember from the previous page.

rose

seeds

tree

water

bush

sand

table

Lovely Words

Word One

Take some time to memorize the word below. Then turn the page and circle the word you remember.

bed

turn the page

Word Two

Take some time to memorize the word below. Then turn the page and circle the word you remember.

milk

turn the page

Memory Game

Puzzle continued from the previous page.

Word One

Circle the word you remember from the previous page.

paint brick cabinet

t-shirt mouse

bed fish

Word Two

Circle the word you remember from the previous page.

window tile

coat milk

paint book yellow

Lovely Words

Word One

Take some time to memorize the word below. Then turn the page and circle the word you remember.

dog

turn the page

Word Two

Take some time to memorize the word below. Then turn the page and circle the word you remember.

pear

turn the page

Memory Game

Puzzle continued from the previous page.

Word One

Circle the word you remember from the previous page.

grass eggs blue

valley dog

table lake

Word Two

Circle the word you remember from the previous page.

oven town

curtains bear

game

pear door

Lovely Words

Word One

Take some time to memorize the word below. Then turn the page and circle the word you remember.

phone

turn the page

Word Two

Take some time to memorize the word below. Then turn the page and circle the word you remember.

bread

turn the page

Memory Game

Puzzle continued from the previous page.

Word One

Circle the word you remember from the previous page.

rose pencil phone

sugar lamp

cards kettle

Word Two

Circle the word you remember from the previous page.

dishes street

bread tiger

raccoon

butter fence

Section Six

Fun Puzzles

MAZES

HOW TO PLAY

MAZES

1. Take a look at the maze.

2. Draw the path that takes you from the start to the finish.

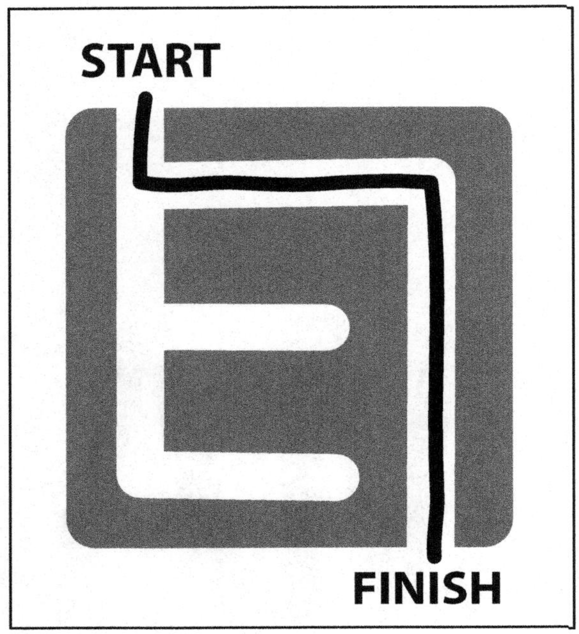

HELPFUL HINTS!

✓ If you cannot find a path that goes from start to finish, try going backwards! Sometimes, if you begin at the finish point and look for a path that goes to the starting point, you will be able to solve the maze.

✓ Take your time solving each maze. If you get stuck, you can always skip a puzzle, and come back to it later.

MAZE

FIND THE PATH THAT GOES FROM START TO FINISH

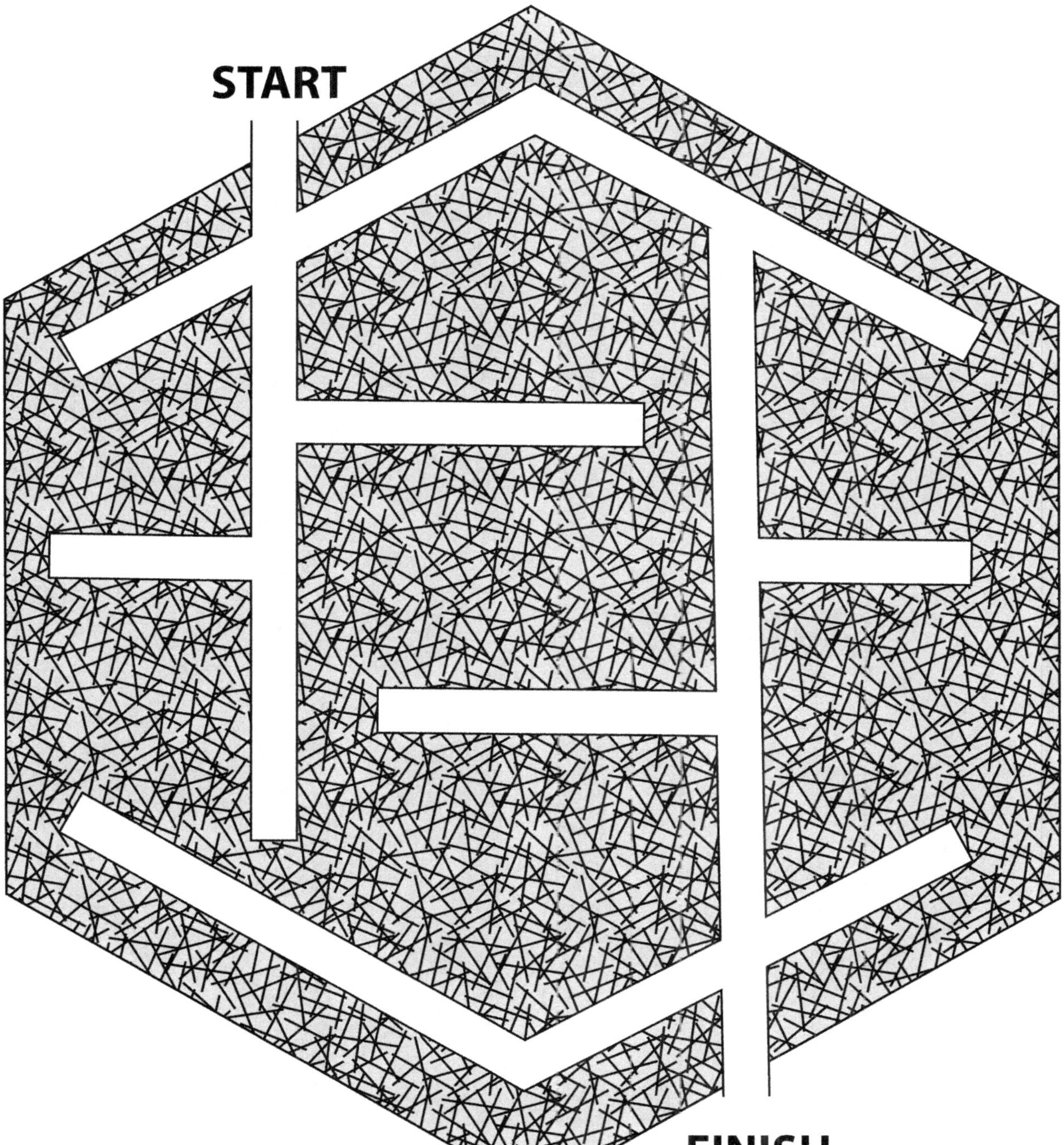

MAZE

FIND THE PATH THAT GOES FROM START TO FINISH

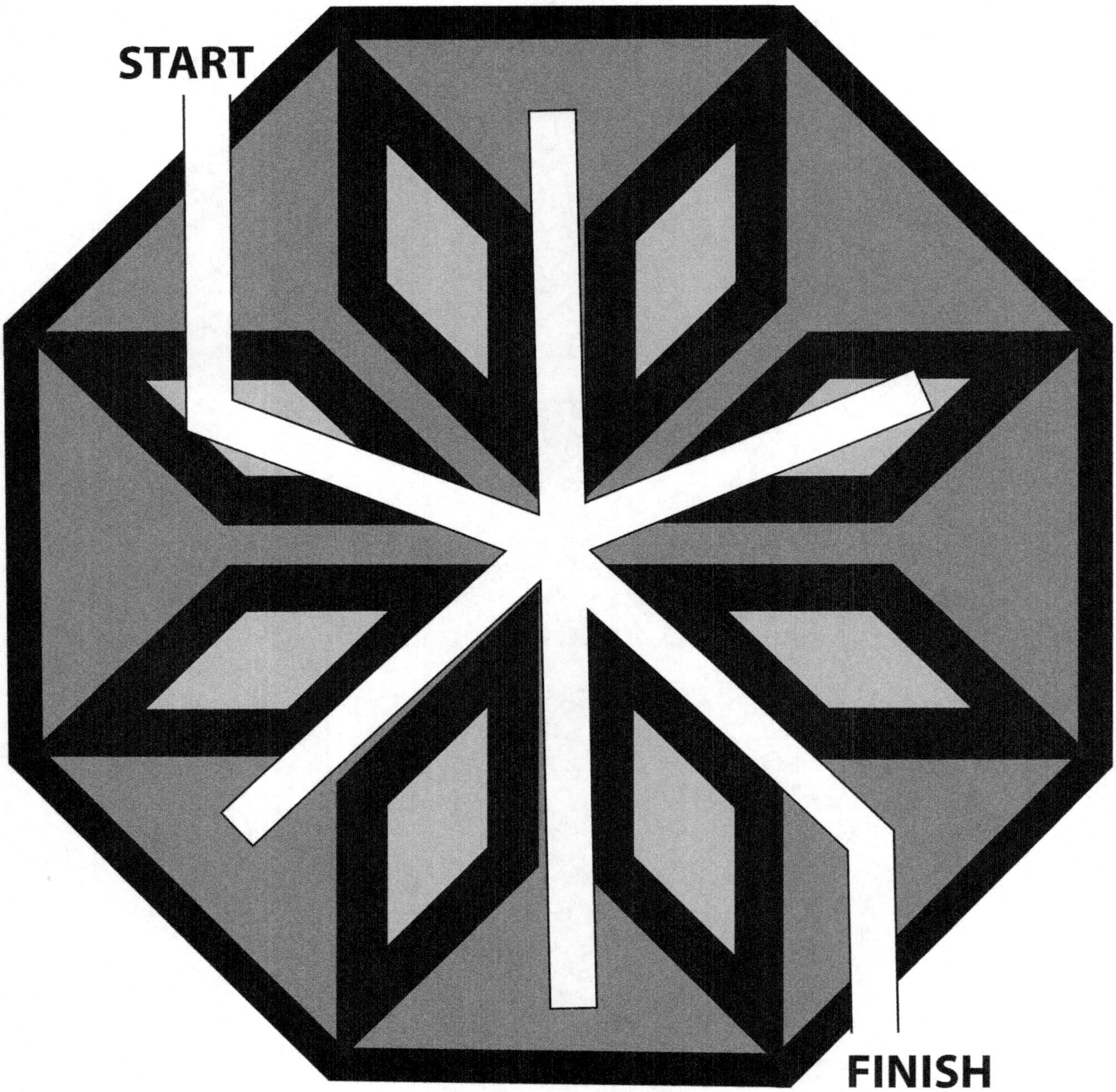

MAZE

FIND THE PATH THAT GOES FROM START TO FINISH

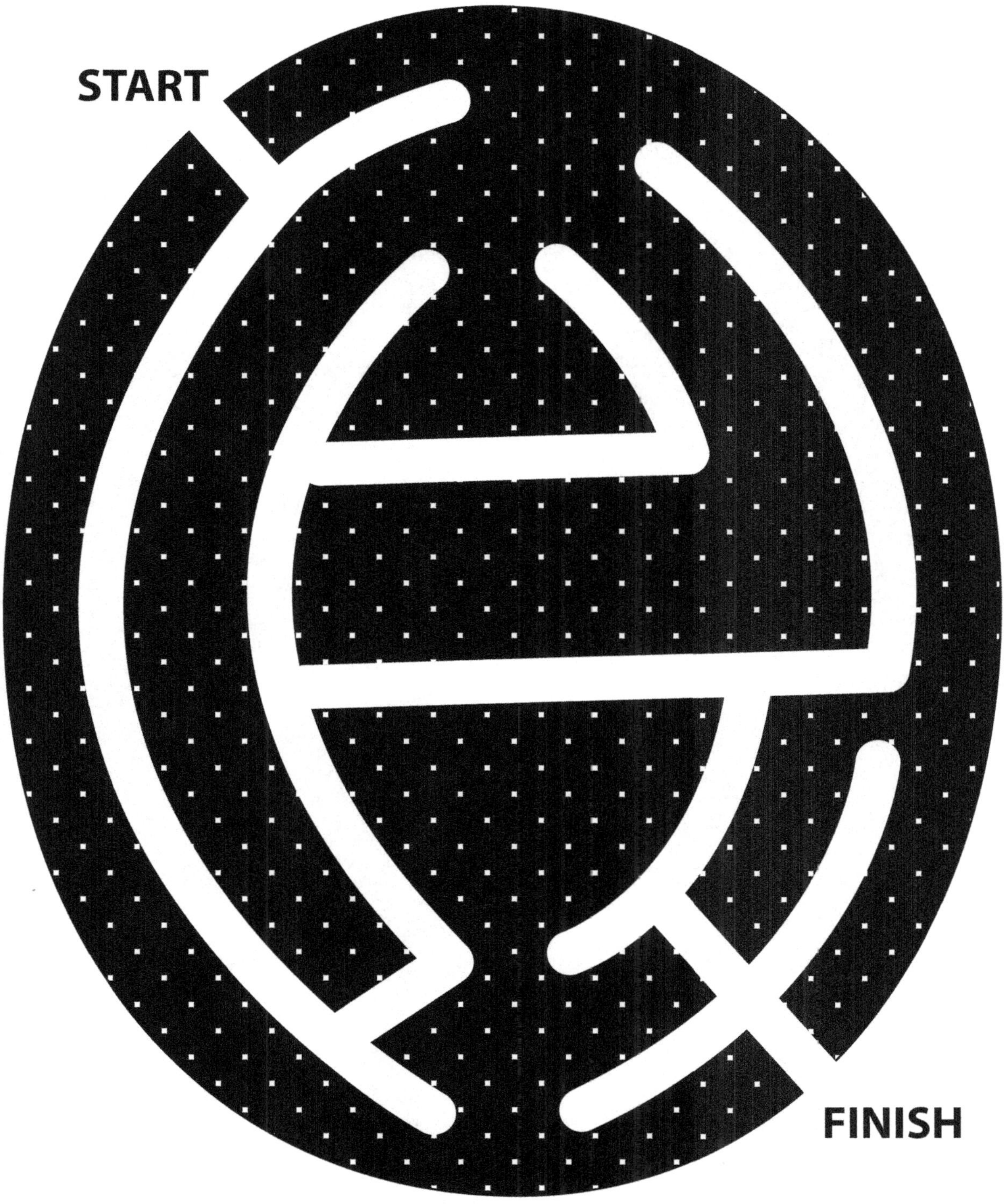

Instructions

MAZE

FIND THE PATH THAT GOES FROM START TO FINISH

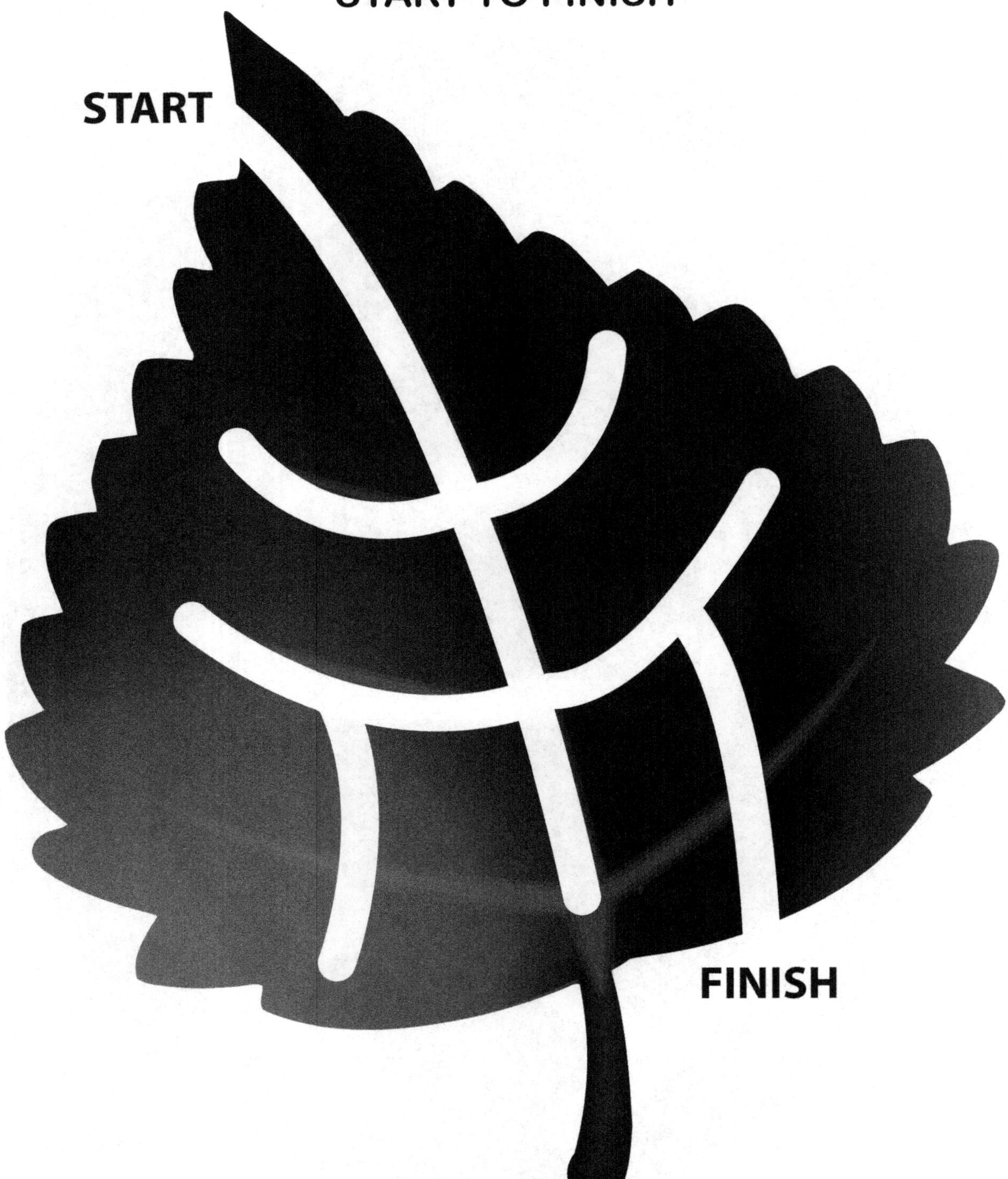

MAZE

FIND THE PATH THAT GOES FROM START TO FINISH

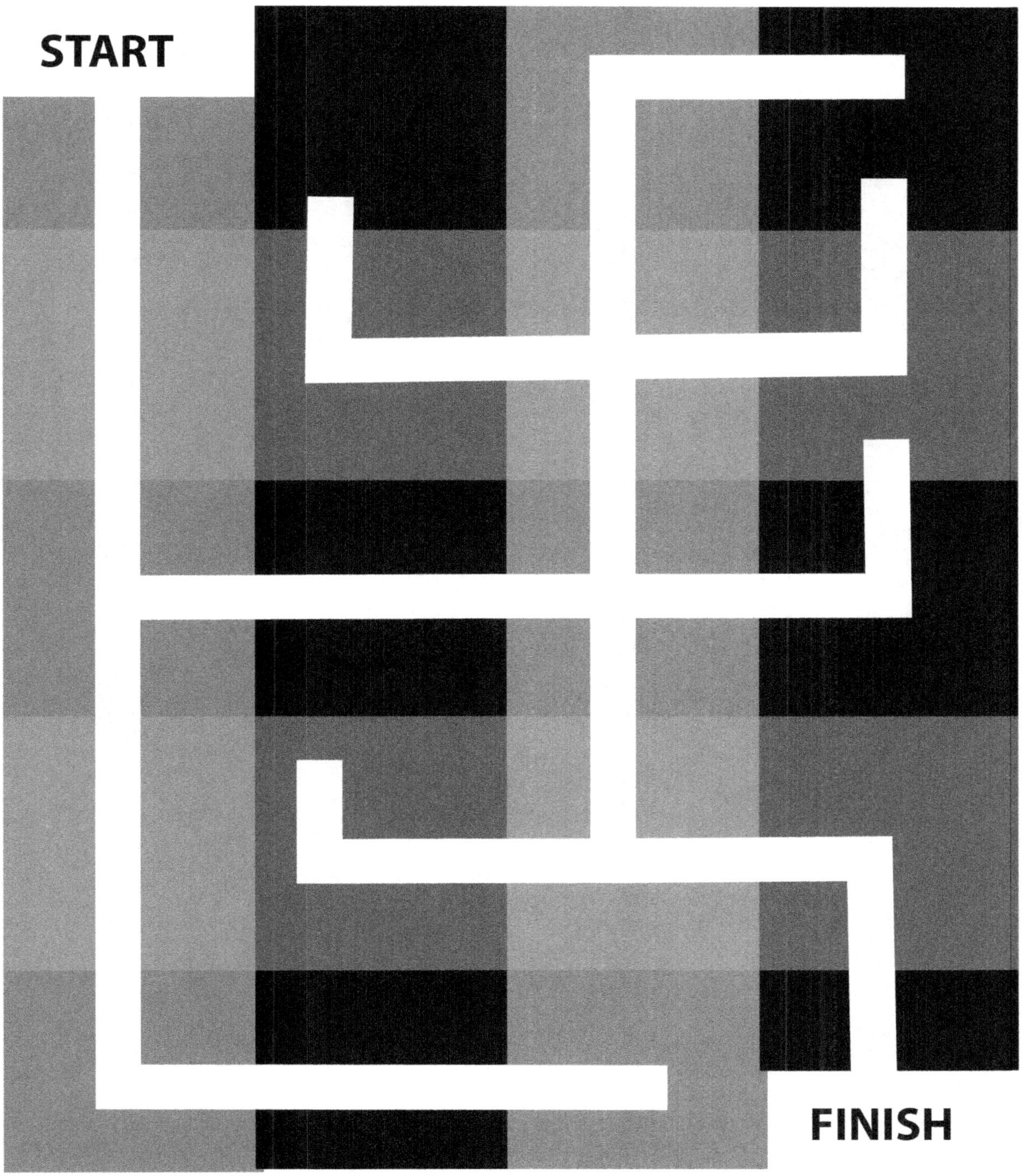

MAZE

FIND THE PATH THAT GOES FROM
START TO FINISH

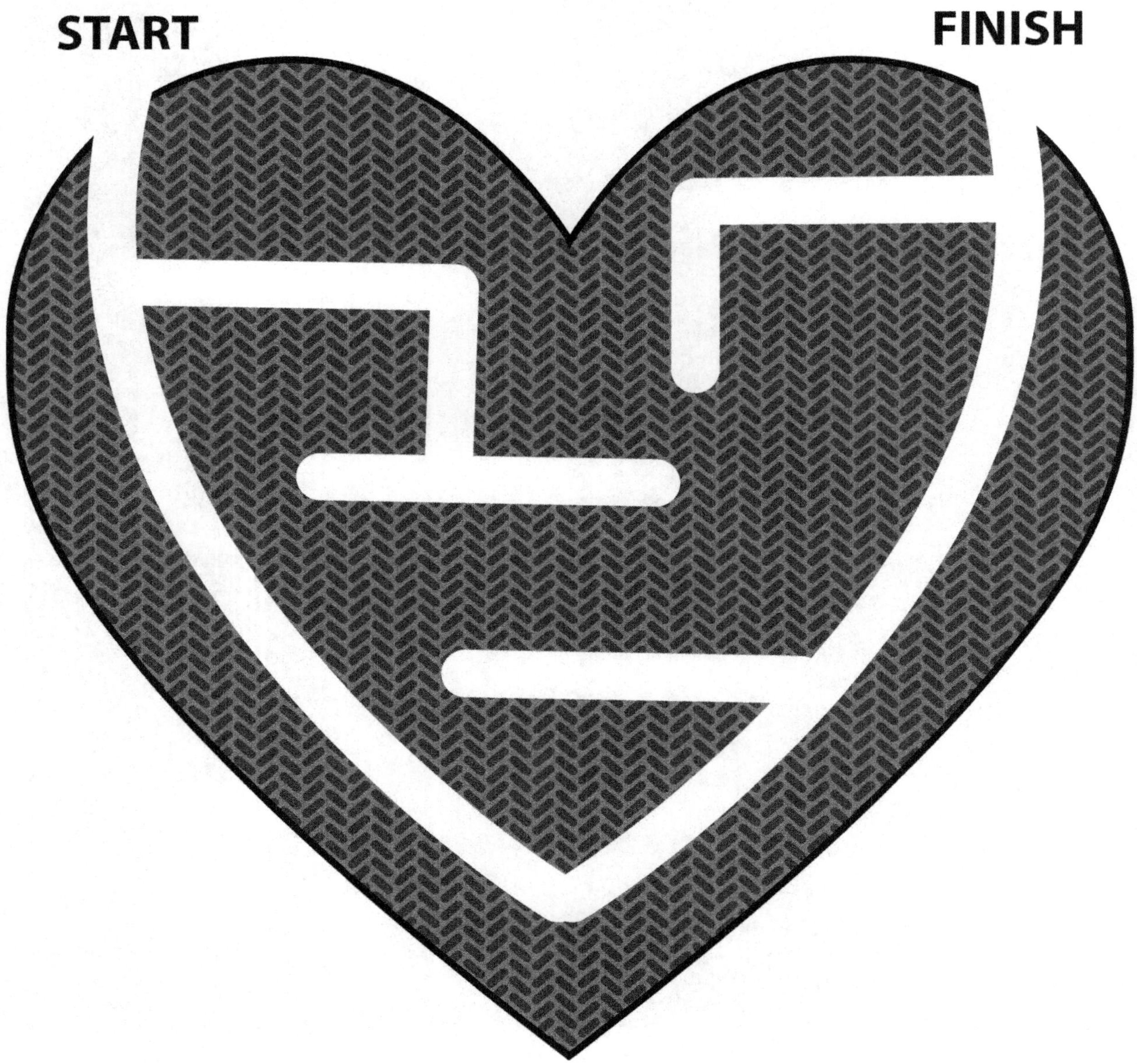

MAZE

FIND THE PATH THAT GOES FROM
START TO FINISH

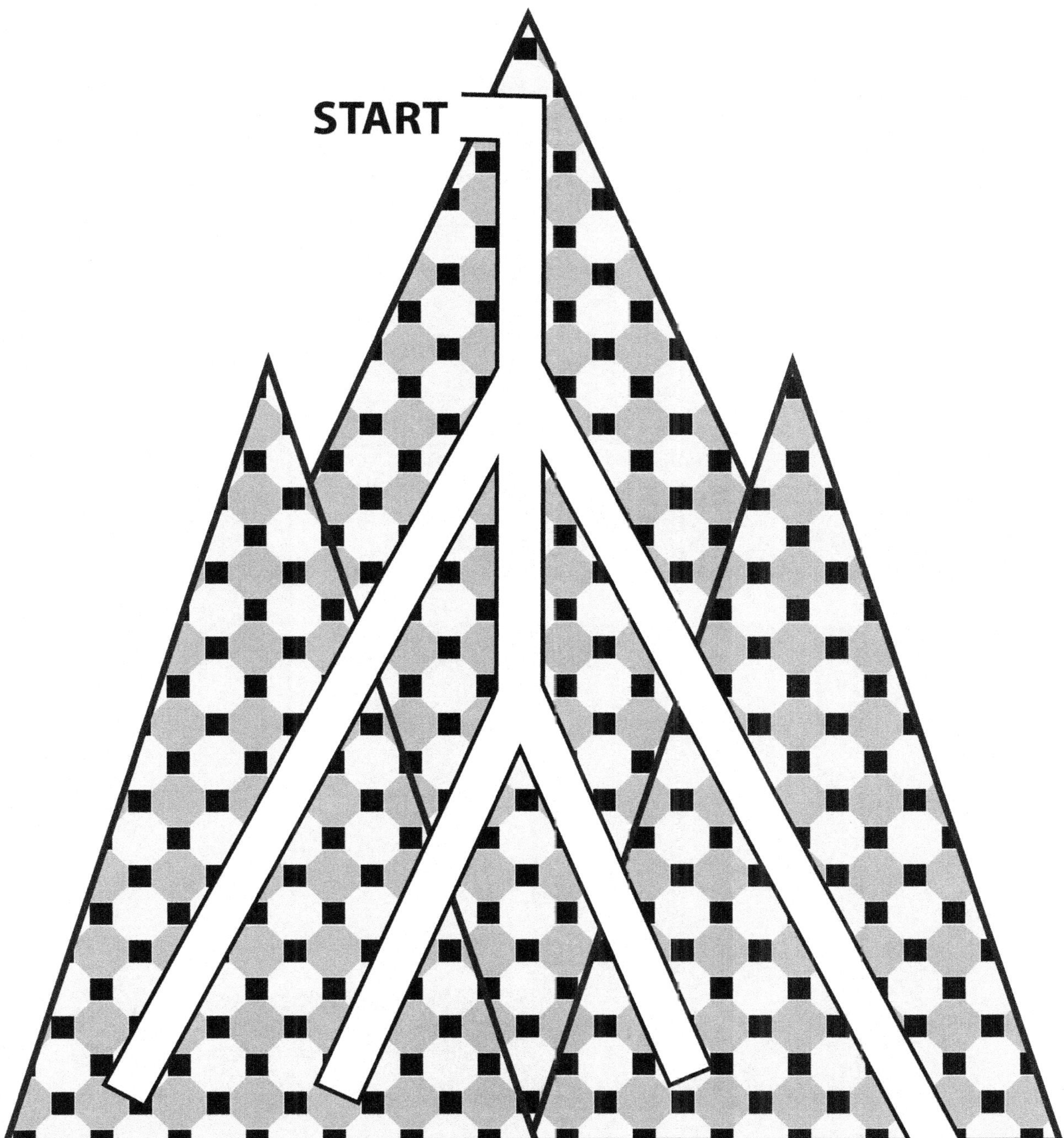

MAZE

FIND THE PATH THAT GOES FROM START TO FINISH

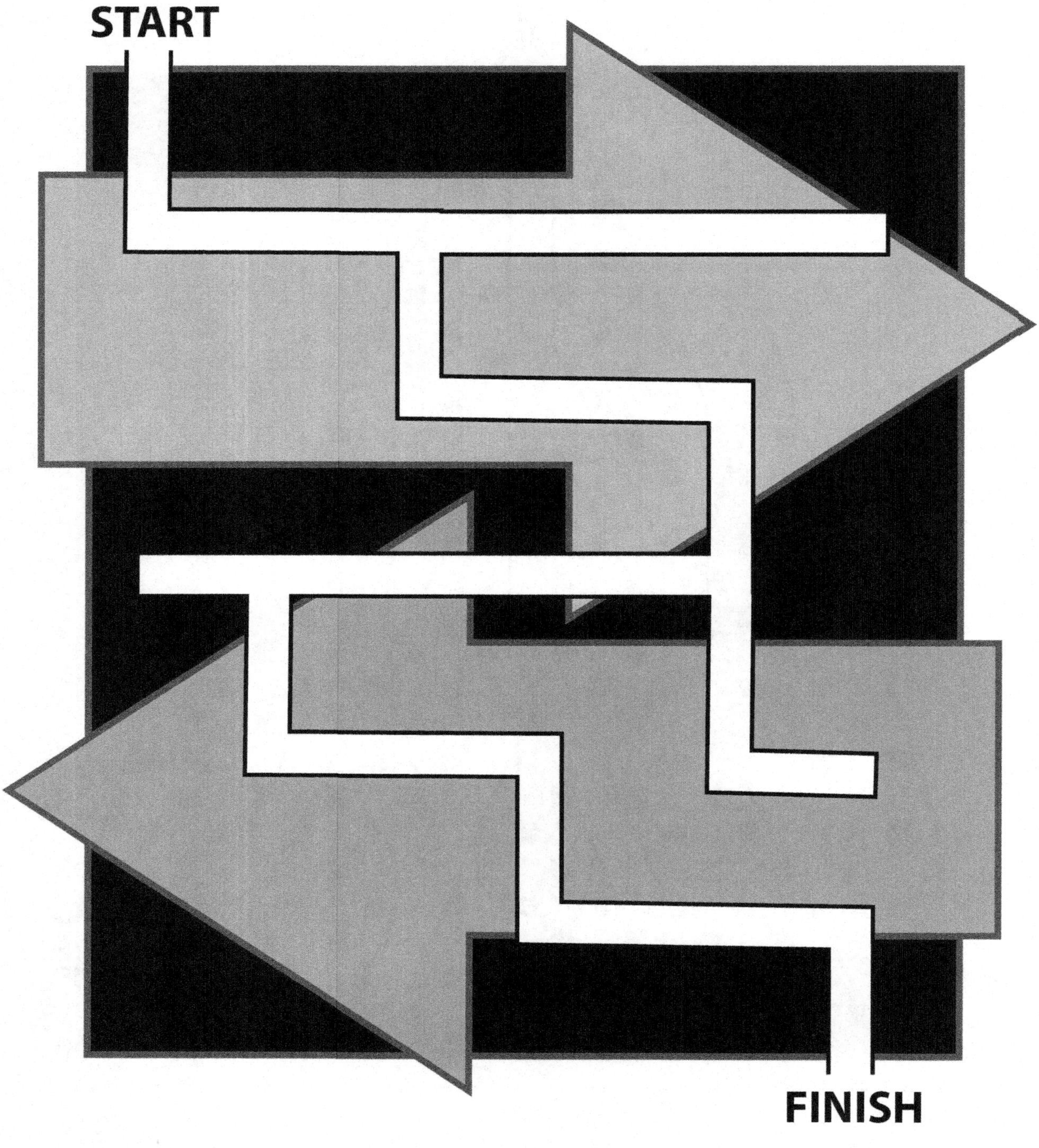

MAZE

FIND THE PATH THAT GOES FROM START TO FINISH

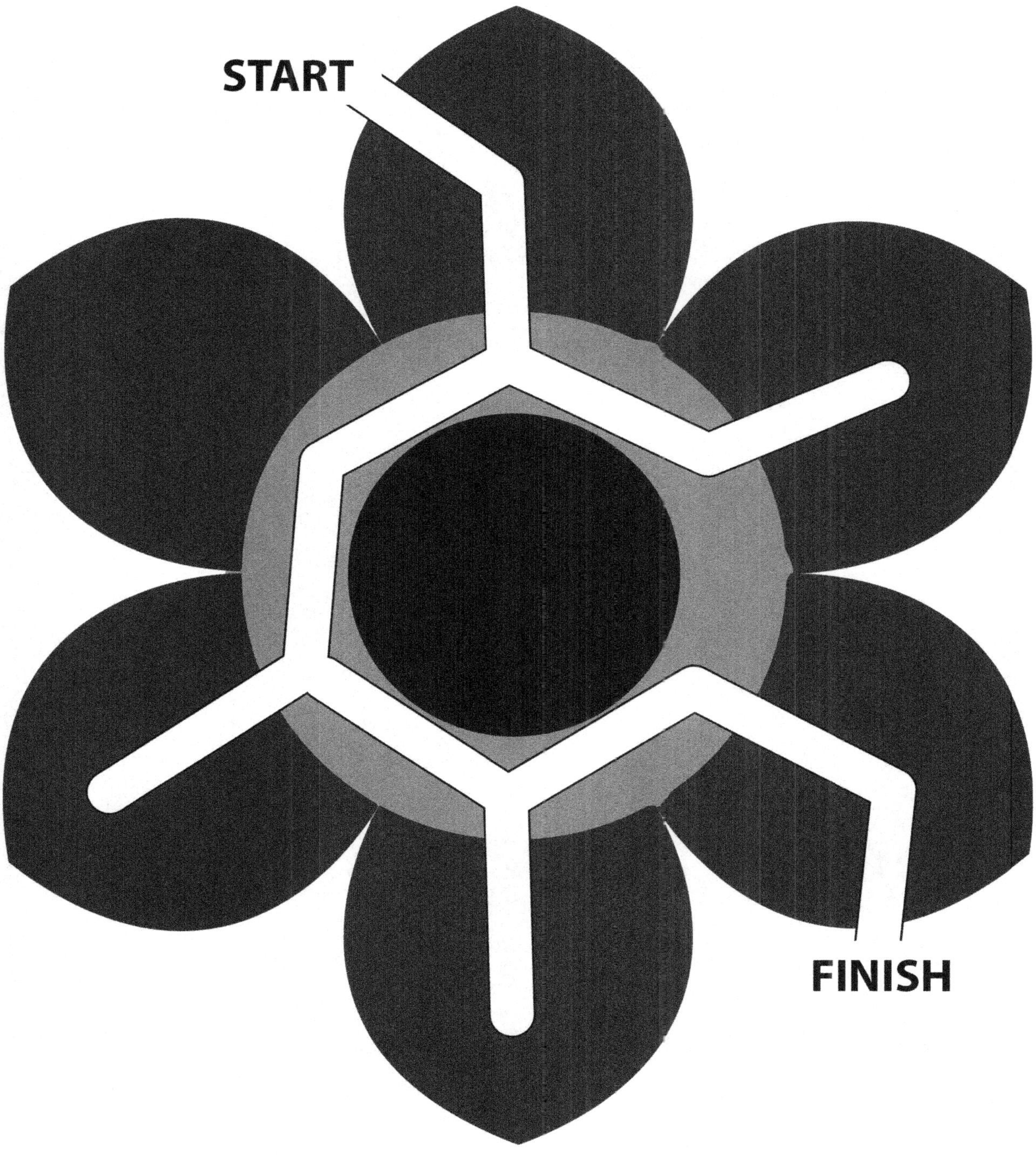

MAZE

FIND THE PATH THAT GOES FROM START TO FINISH

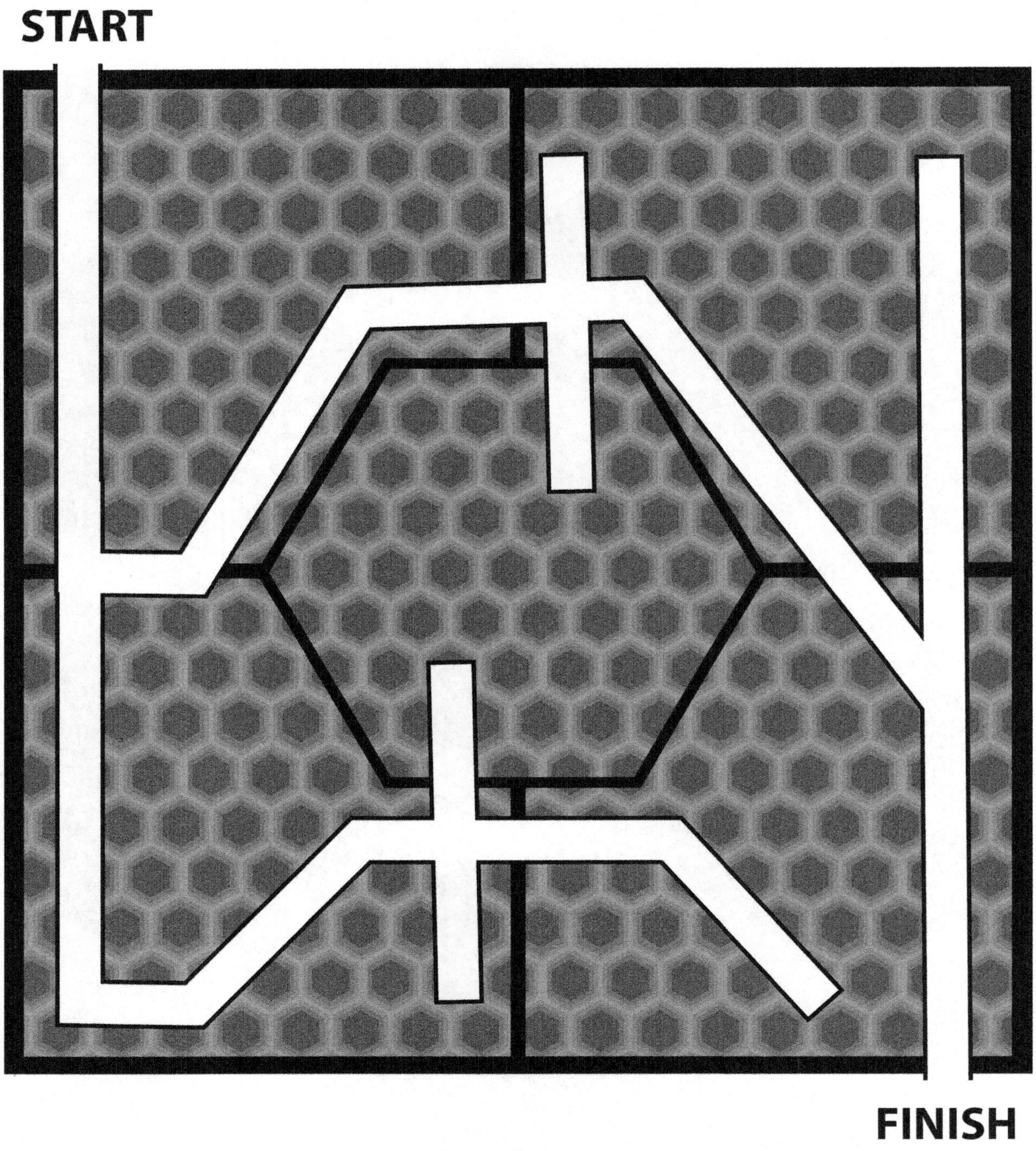

MAZE

FIND THE PATH THAT GOES FROM START TO FINISH

Fun Puzzle

MAZE

FIND THE PATH THAT GOES FROM START TO FINISH

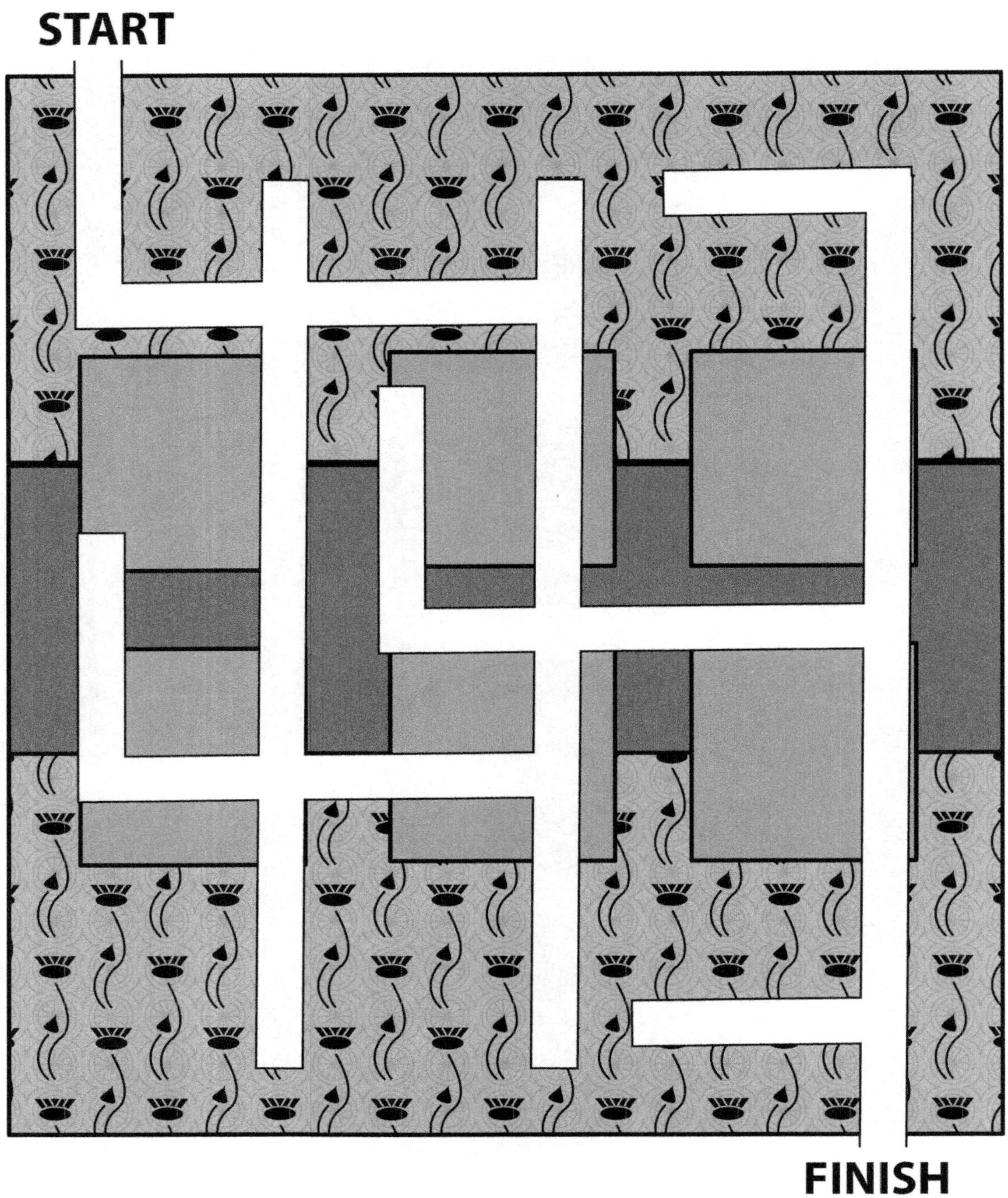

Section Seven

Fun Puzzles & Memory Games

BONUS ACTIVITIES

Fun Puzzle

FIND 3 DIFFERENCES

FIND THE THREE DIFFERENCES BETWEEN THE TWO PICTURES

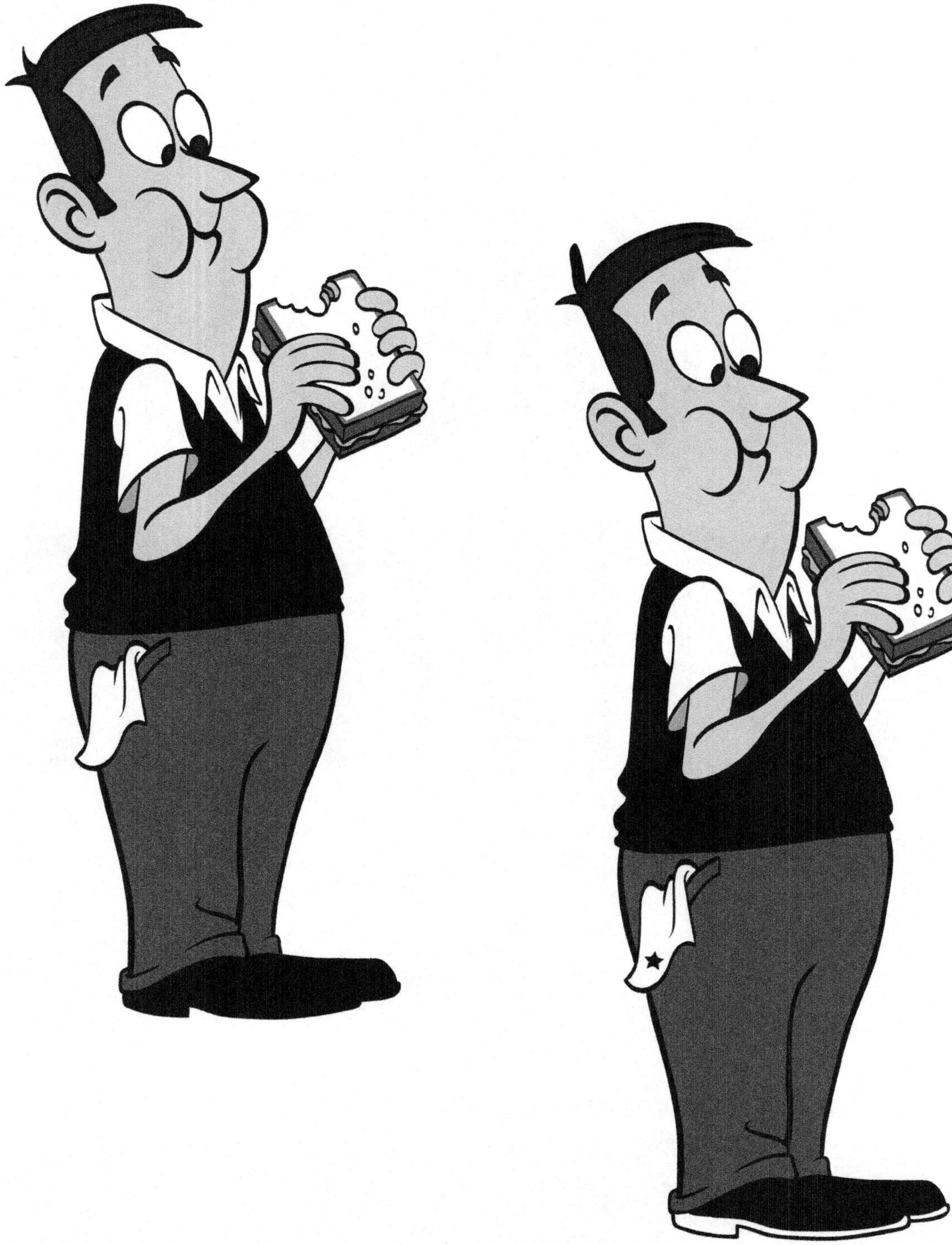

Fun Puzzle

Favorite Number

Harry's favorite number is:

12

Memorize the number above. Then turn the page, and pick out the number from a selection of numbers.

turn the page

Jen's favorite number is:

28

Memorize the number above. Then turn the page, and pick out the number from a selection of numbers.

turn the page

Fun Puzzle

Puzzle continued from the previous page.

Which number is Harry's favorite?

Circle the number that you remember from the previous page.

71 43

52 12

Which number is Jen's favorite?

Circle the number that you remember from the previous page.

28 51

14 20

MAZE

FIND THE PATH THAT GOES FROM START TO FINISH

START

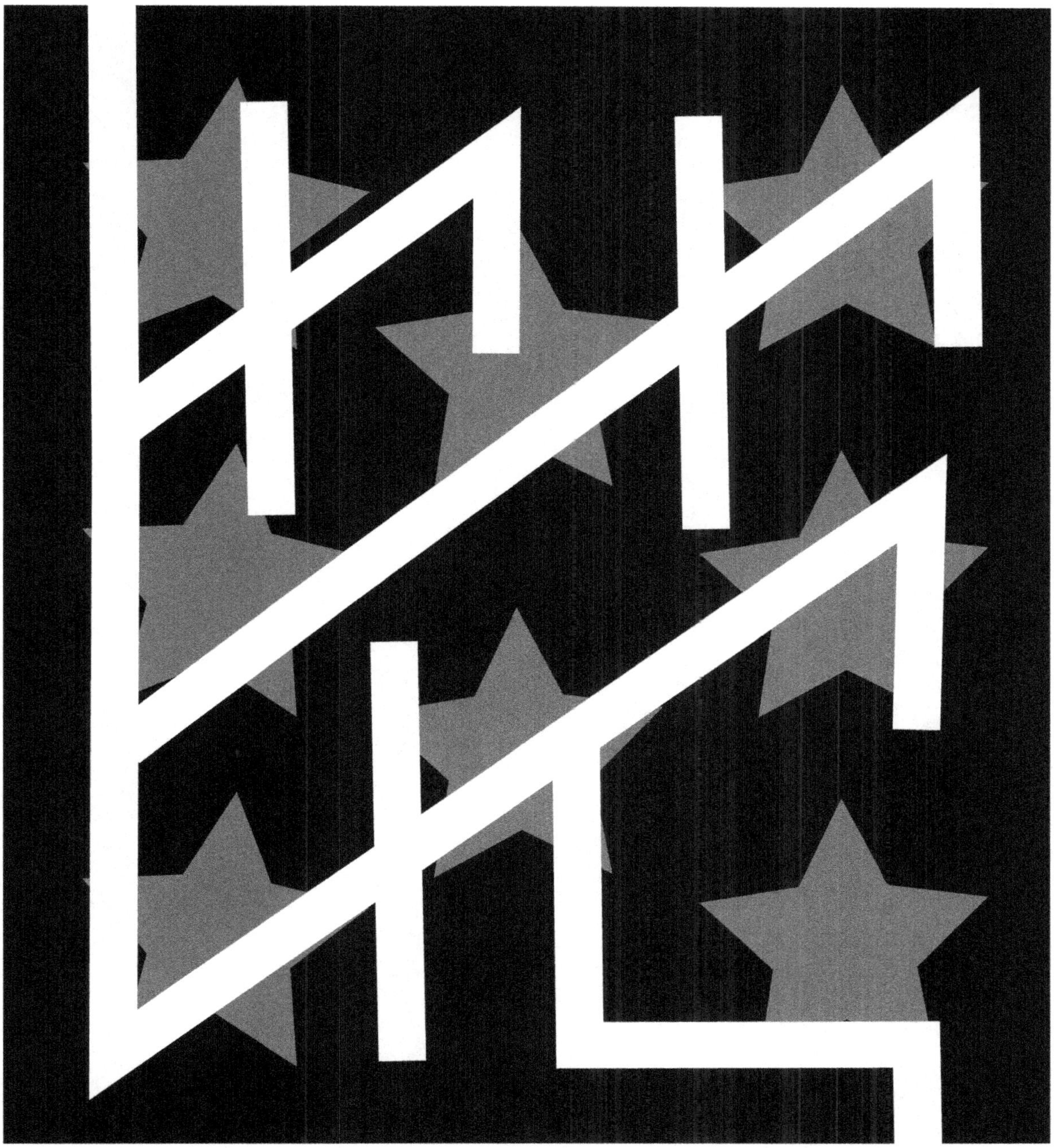

FINISH

Fun Puzzle

SPOT THE ODD ONE OUT

FIND THE MOUSE THAT IS DIFFERENT FROM THE REST

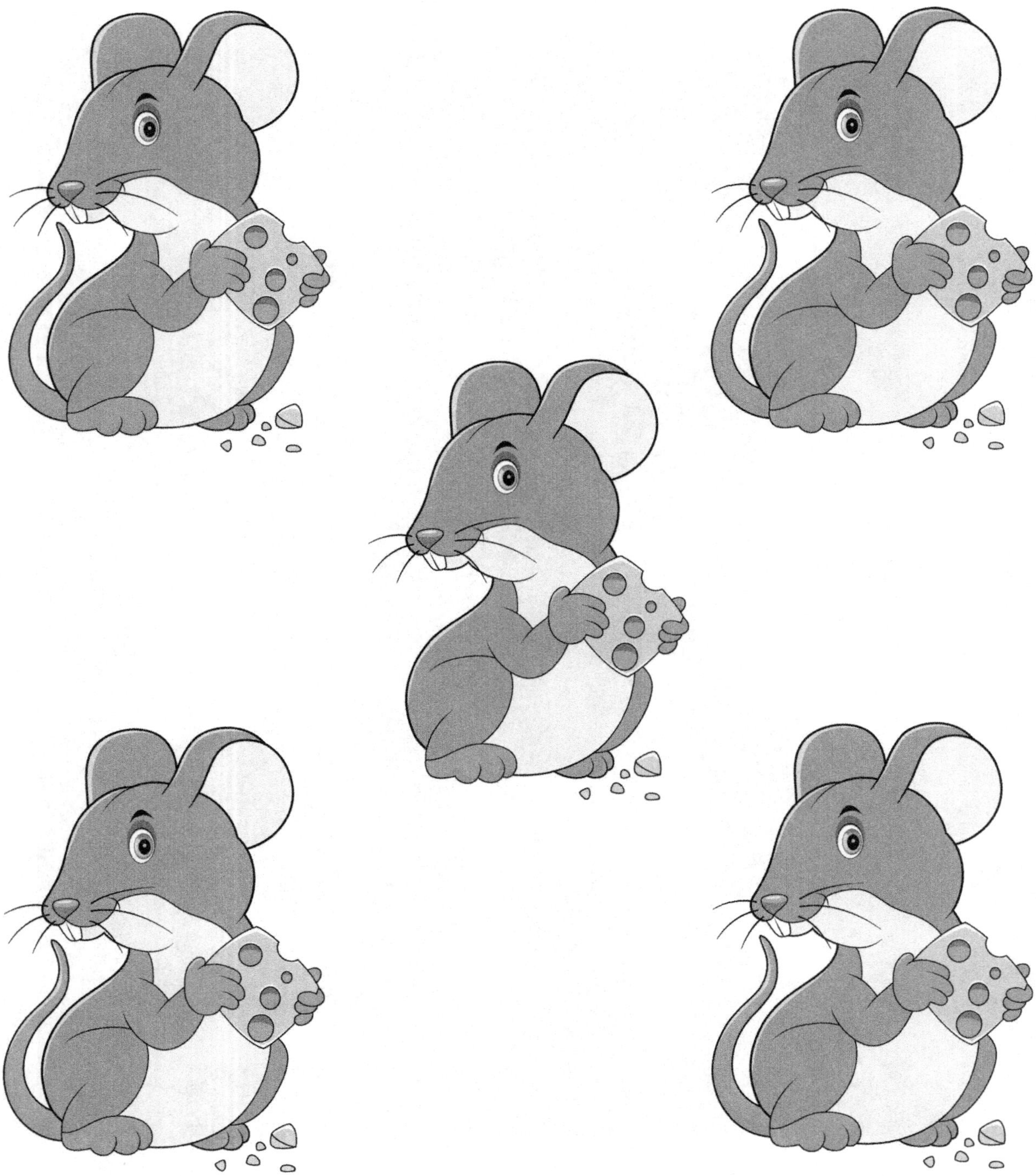

Fun Puzzle

Lovely Words

Word One

Take some time to memorize the word below. Then turn the page and circle the word you remember.

towel

turn the page

Word Two

Take some time to memorize the word below. Then turn the page and circle the word you remember.

rose

turn the page

Fun Puzzle

Puzzle continued from the previous page.

Word One

Circle the word you remember from the previous page.

tree marker knee

coffee towel

rope plate

Word Two

Circle the word you remember from the previous page.

cup paper

lion

rose maker

television bushes

FIND 3 DIFFERENCES

FIND THE THREE DIFFERENCES BETWEEN THE TWO PICTURES

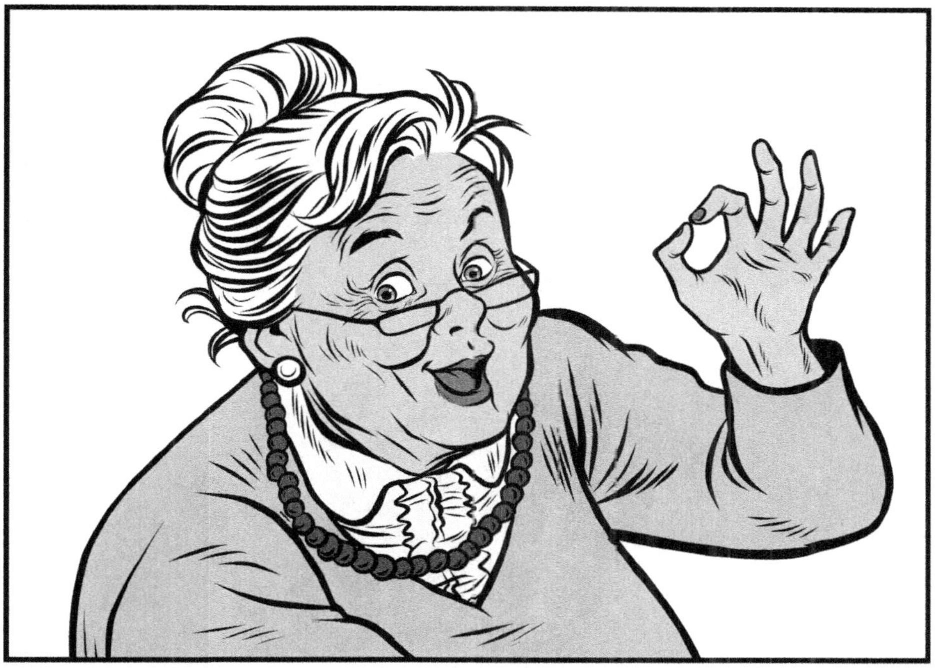

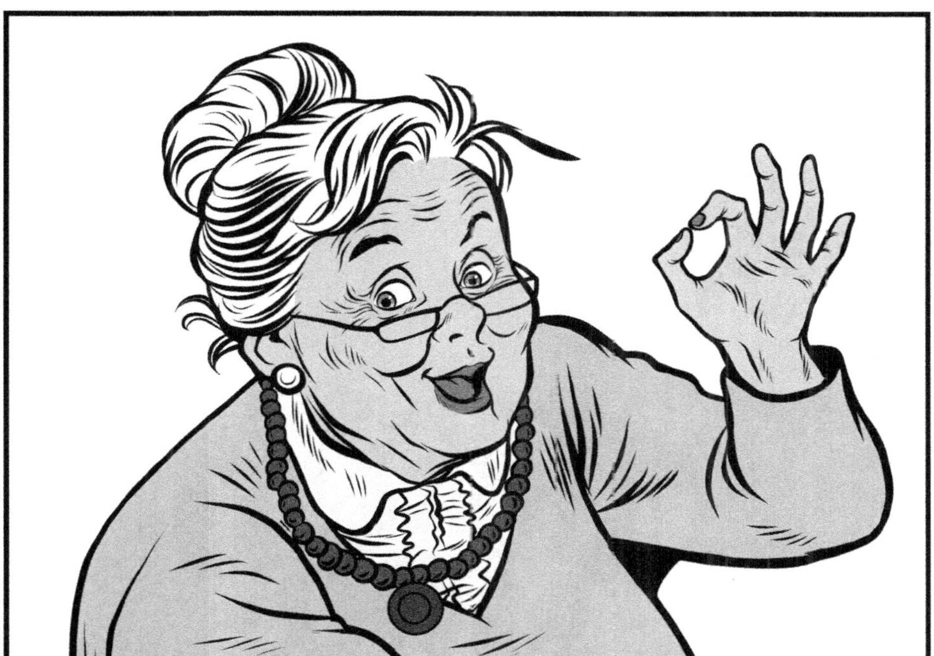

SPOT THE ODD ONE OUT

FIND THE ‘THANK YOU’ THAT IS DIFFERENT FROM THE REST

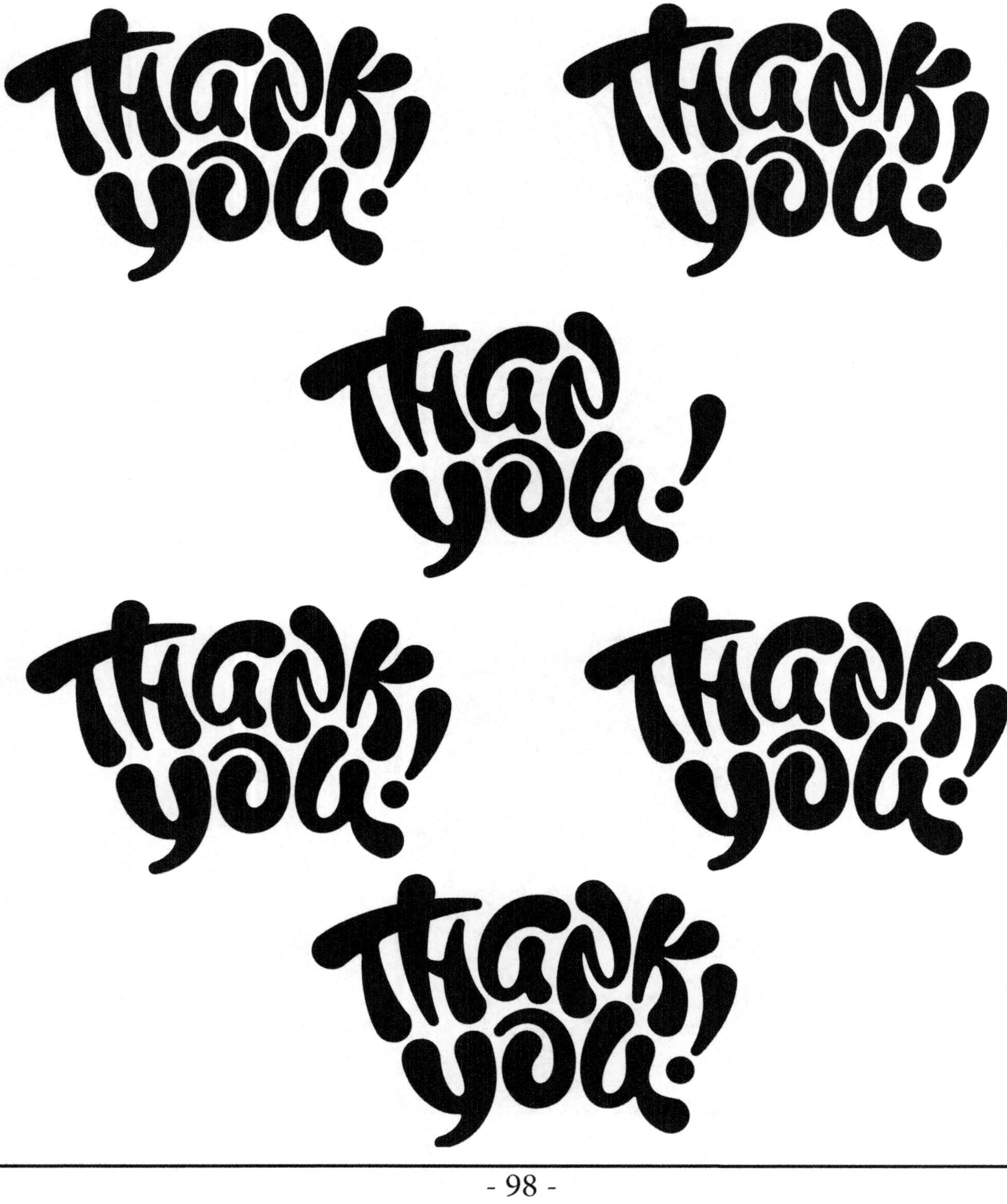

Section Eight

ANSWERS

Answers

Pages 7-8: Picture One

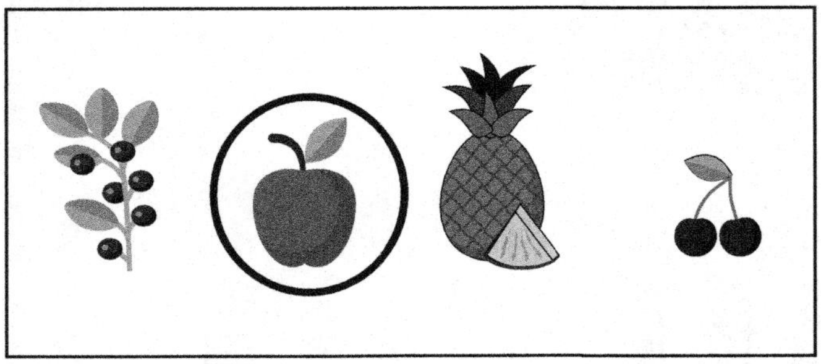

Pages 7-8: Picture Two

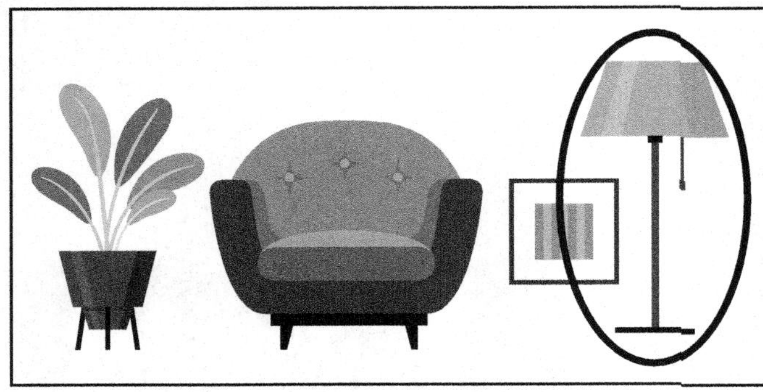

Pages 9-10: Picture One

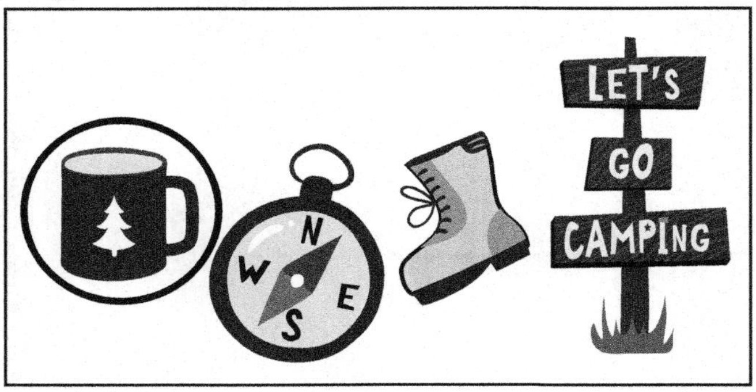

Pages 9-10: Picture Two

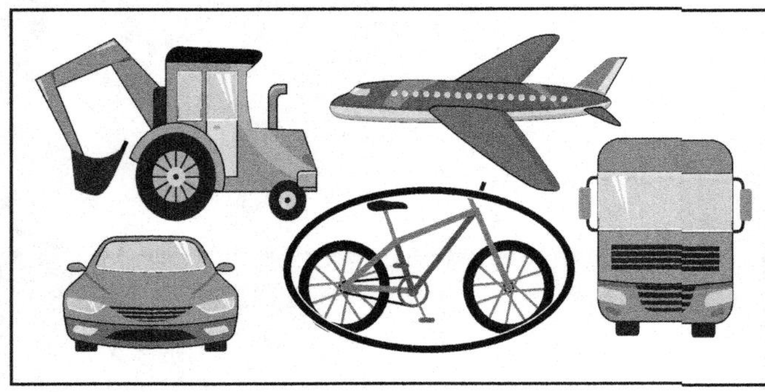

Pages 11-12: Picture One

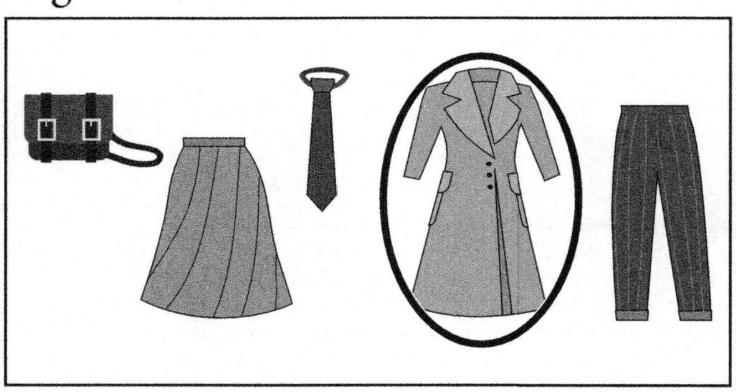

Pages 11-12: Picture Two

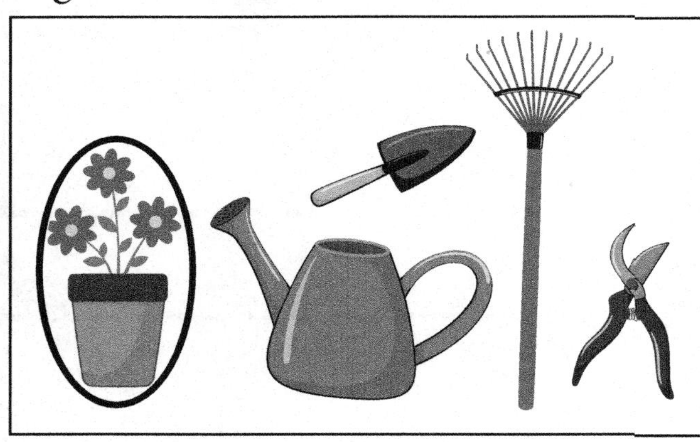

Pages 13-14: Picture One

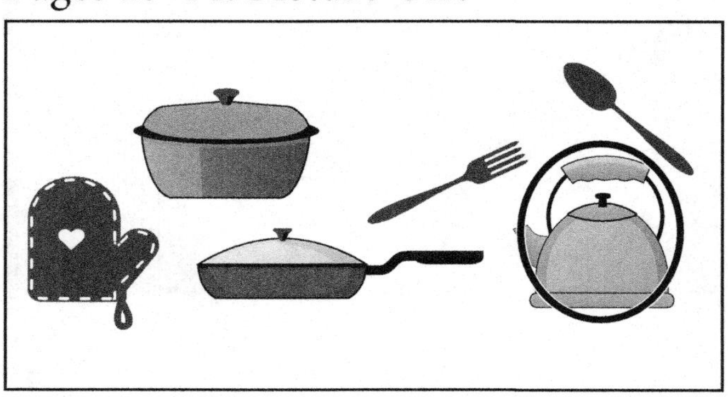

Pages 13-14: Picture Two

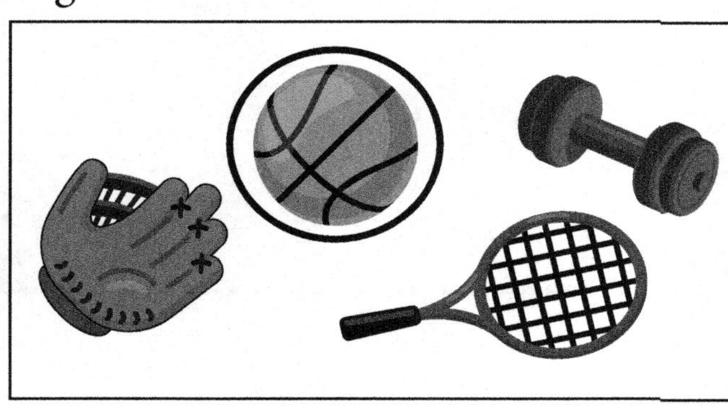

Pages 15-16: Picture One

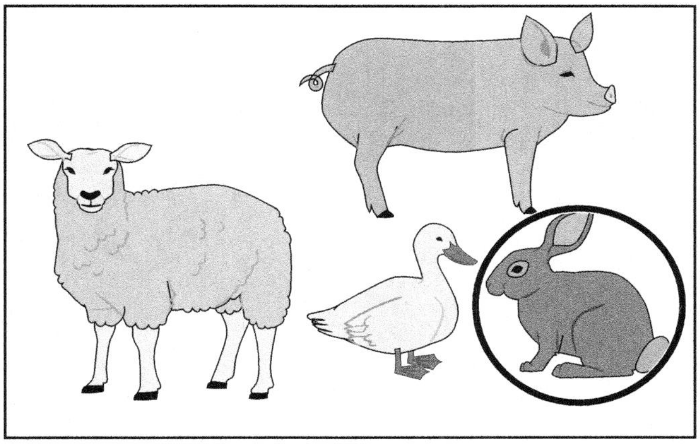

Pages 15-16: Picture Two

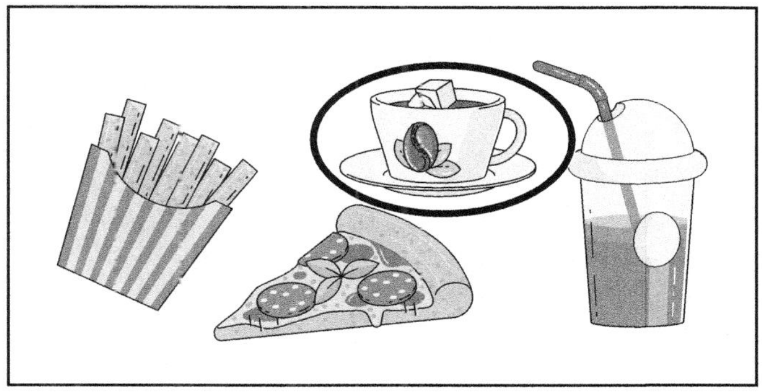

Pages 17-18: Picture One

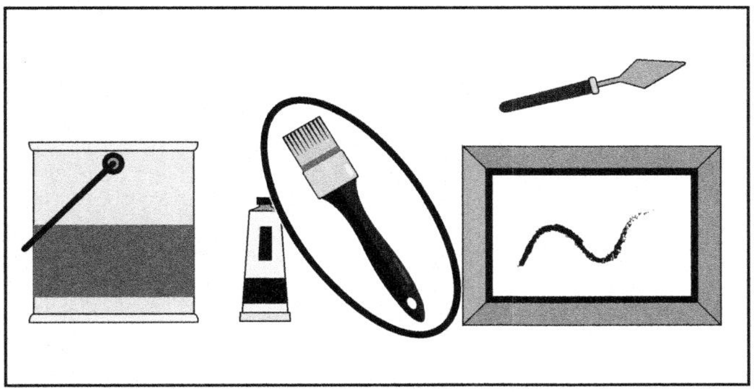

Pages 17-18: Picture Two

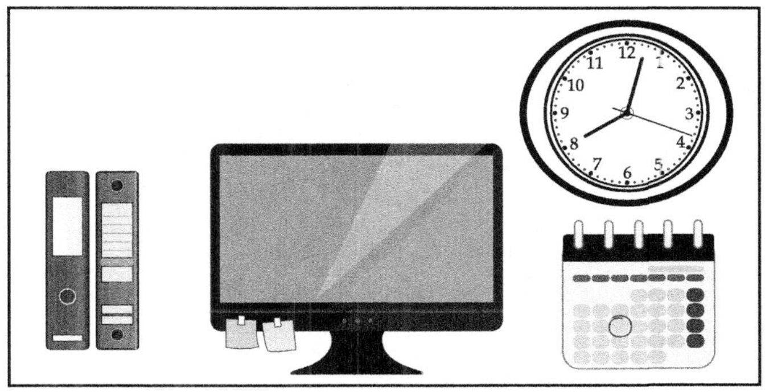

Page 21: Spot the Odd One Out

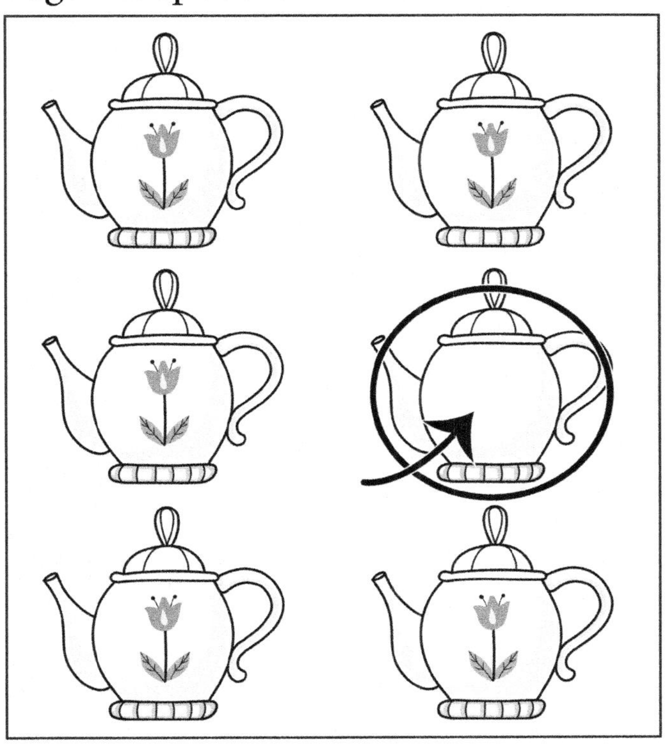

Page 22: Spot the Odd One Out

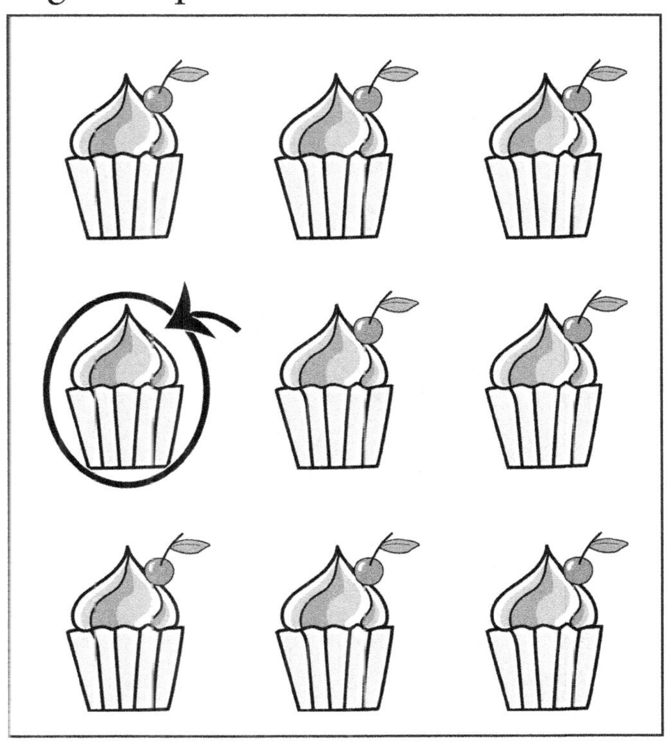

Answers

Page 23: Spot the Odd One Out

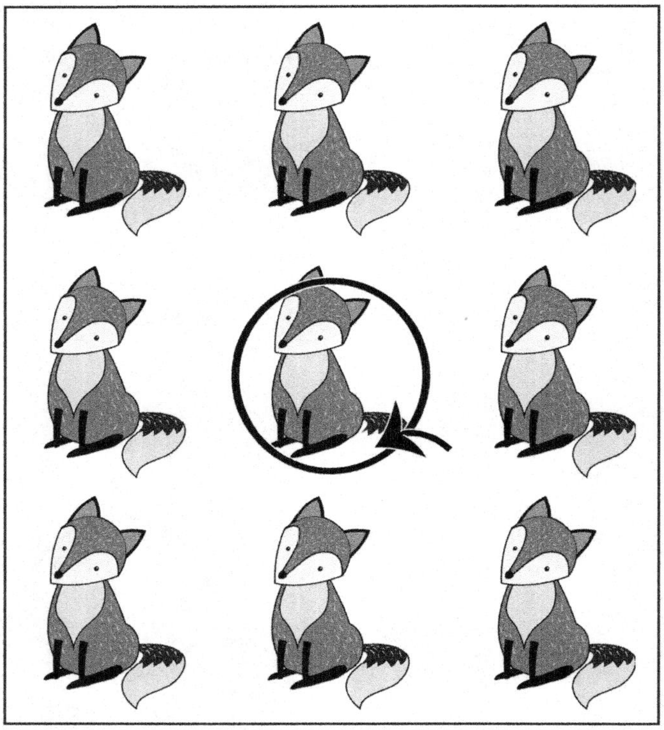

Page 24: Spot the Odd One Out

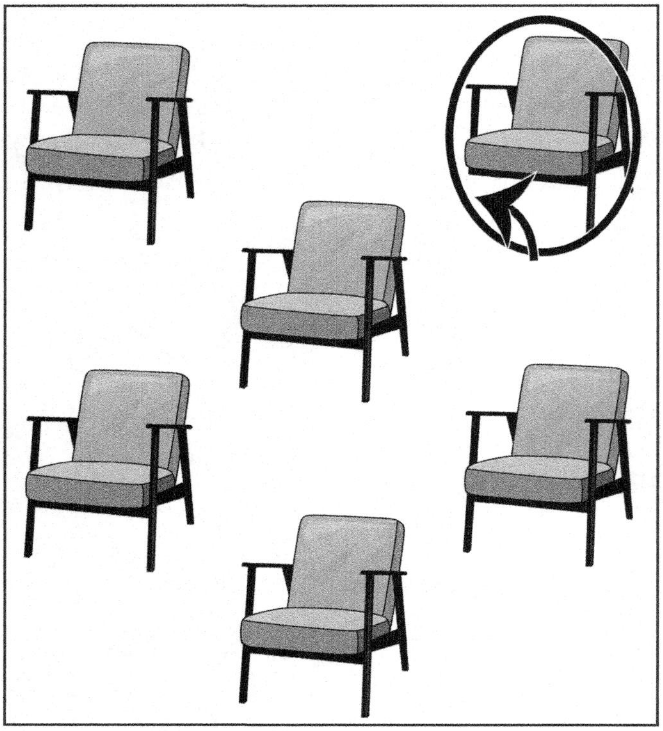

Page 25: Spot the Odd One Out

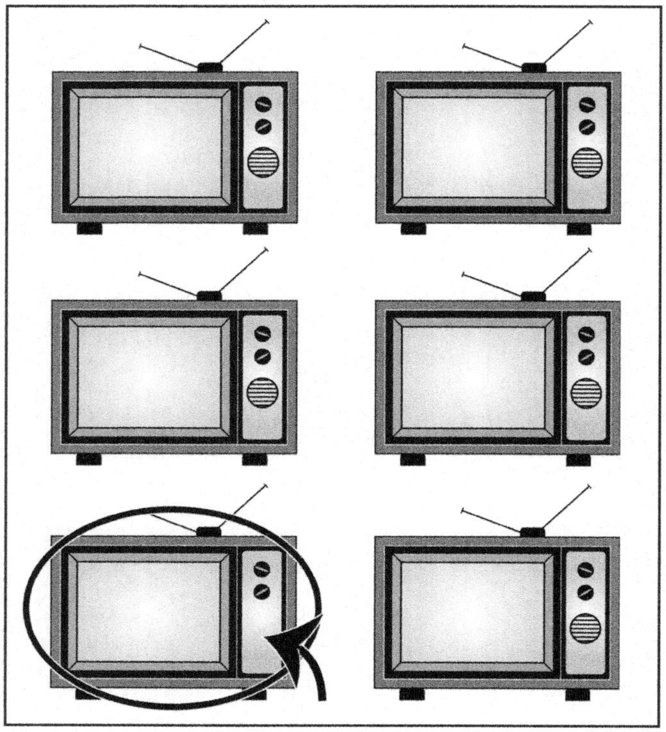

Page 26: Spot the Odd One Out

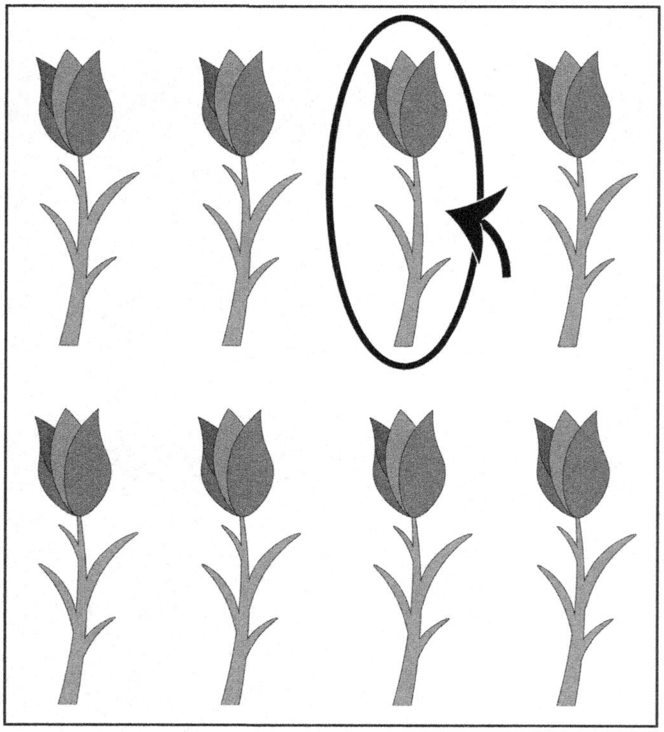

Page 27: Spot the Odd One Out

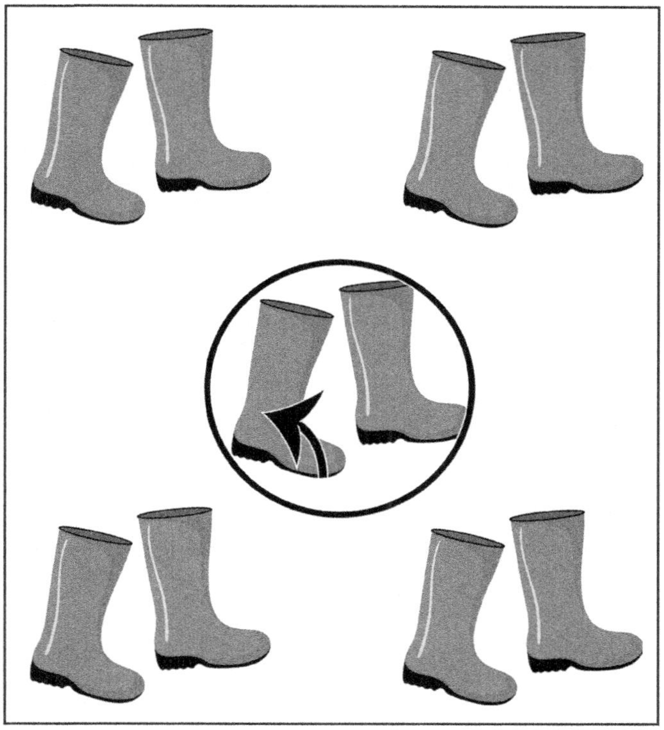

Page 28: Spot the Odd One Out

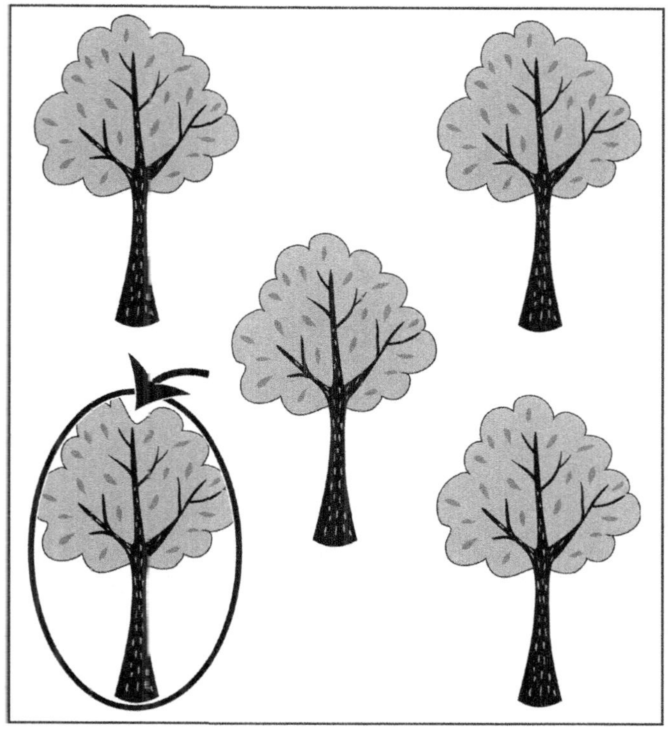

Page 29: Spot the Odd One Out

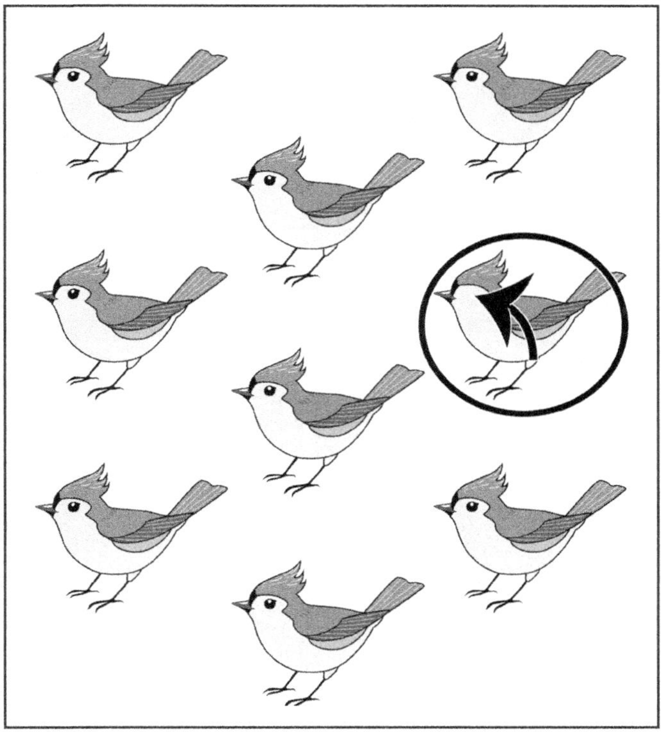

Page 30: Spot the Odd One Out

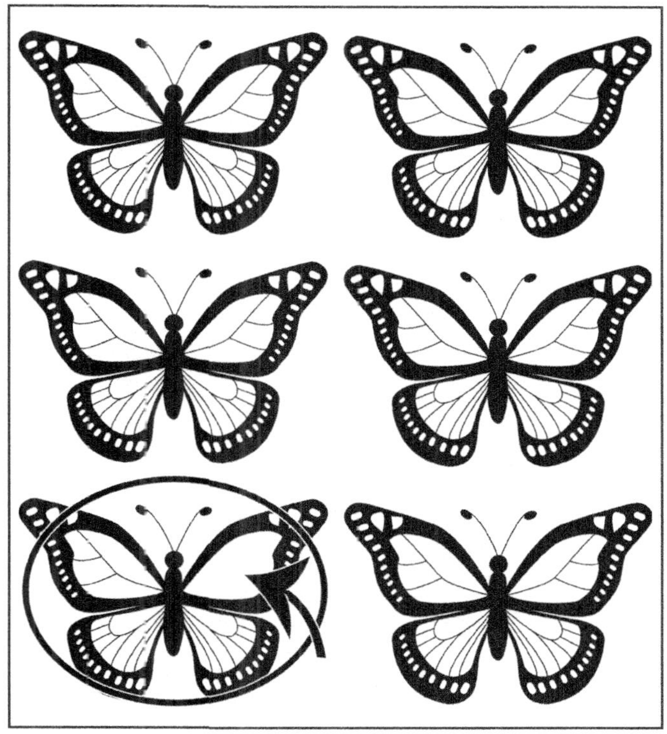

Answers

Page 31: Spot the Odd One Out

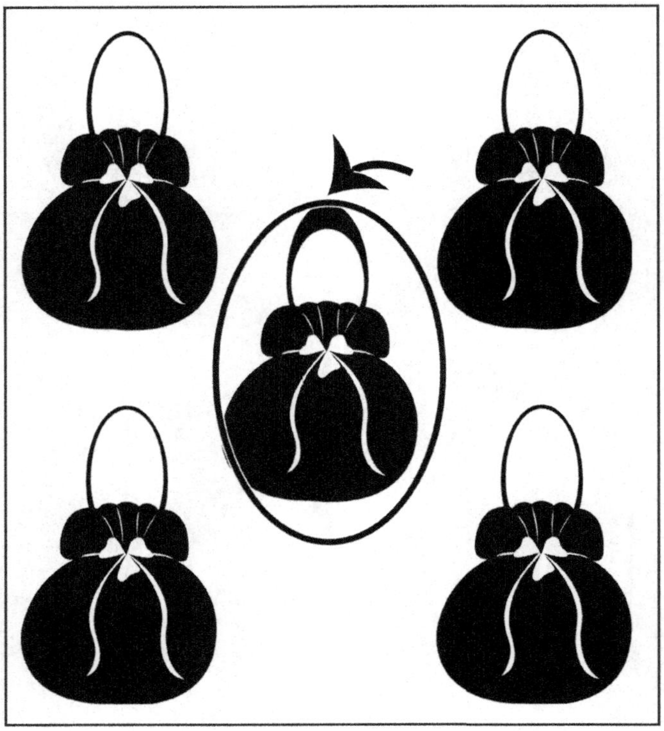

Page 32: Spot the Odd One Out

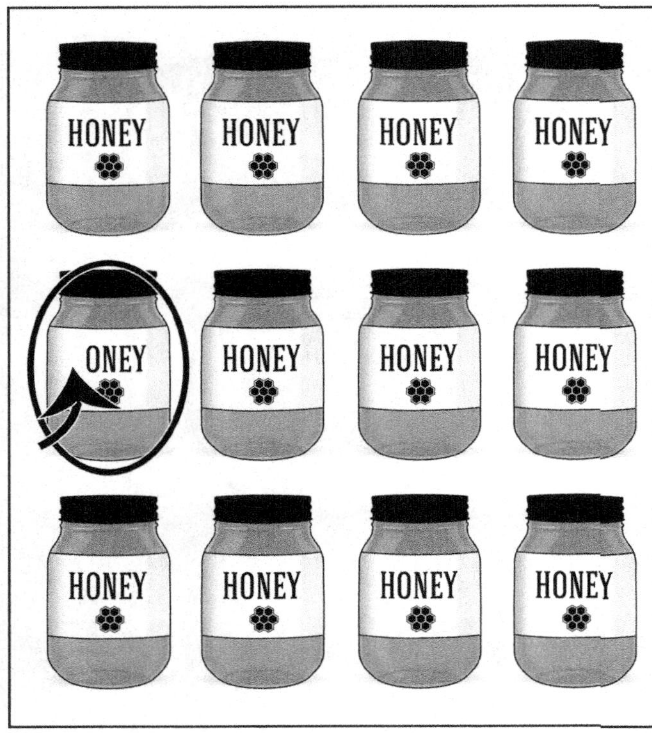

Pages 35-36: Lisa's Favorite Number

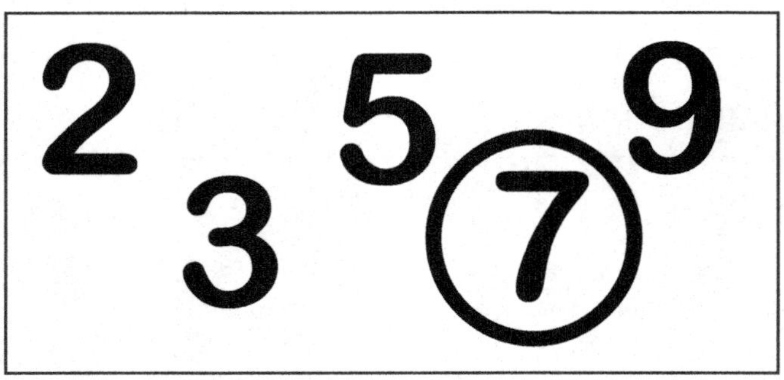

Pages 35-36: Edward's Favorite Num.

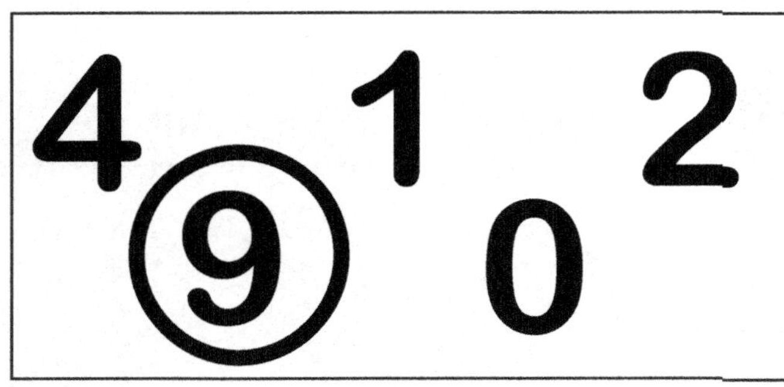

Pages 37-38: John's Favorite Number

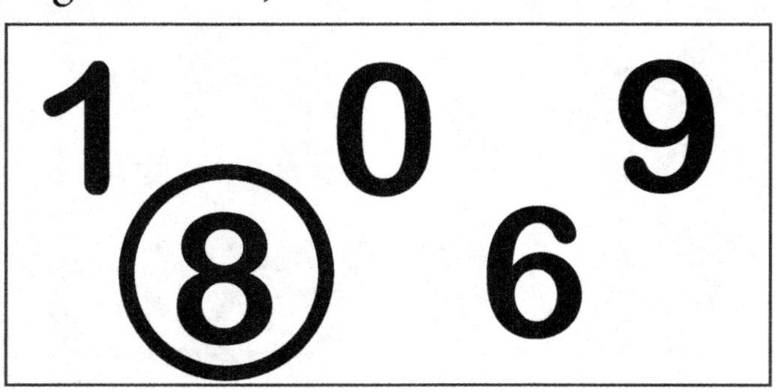

Pages 37-38: Elaine's Favorite Number

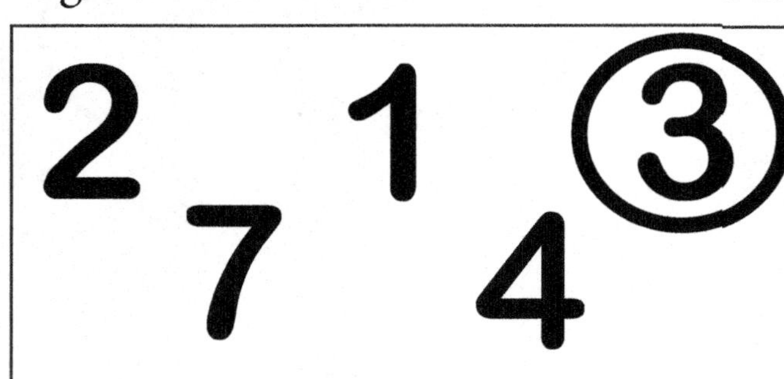

Pages 39-40: Rachel's Favorite Number

7 4 6
2 3

Pages 39-40: William's Favorite Num.

9 5 1
0 2

Pages 41-42: Preston's Favorite Num.

23 46
12 30

Pages 41-42: Larry's Favorite Num.

40 28
32 15

Pages 43-44: Monica's Favorite Num.

32 14
21 53

Pages 43-44: Frasier's Favorite Num.

15 26
30 18

Pages 45-46: Jamie's Favorite Number

51 17
42 25

Pages 45-46: Kate's Favorite Number

37 62
11 29

Answers

Page 49: Find 3 Dif.

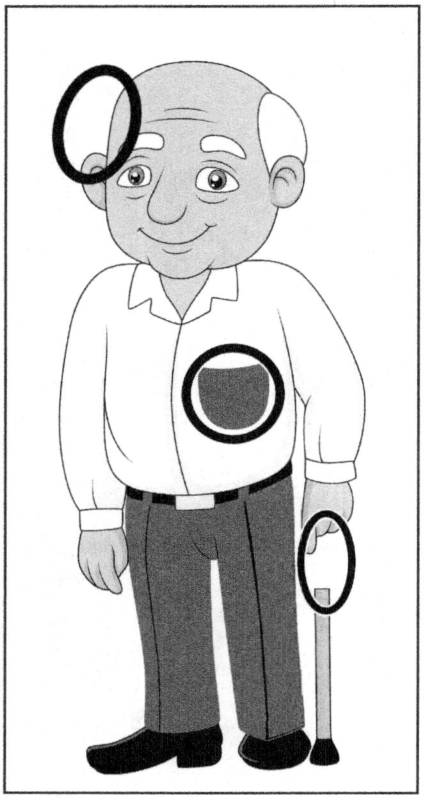

Page 50: Find 3 Dif.

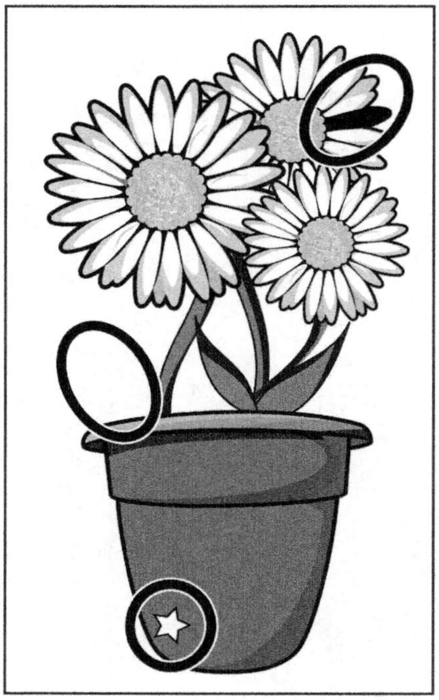

Page 51: Find 3 Dif.

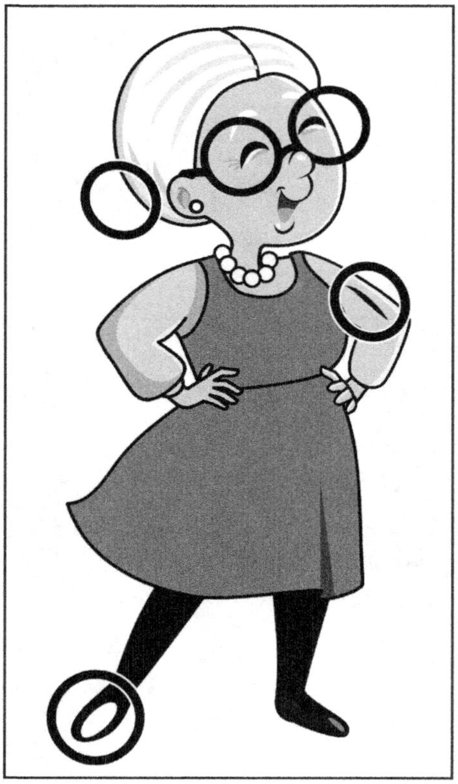

Page 52: Find 3 Differences

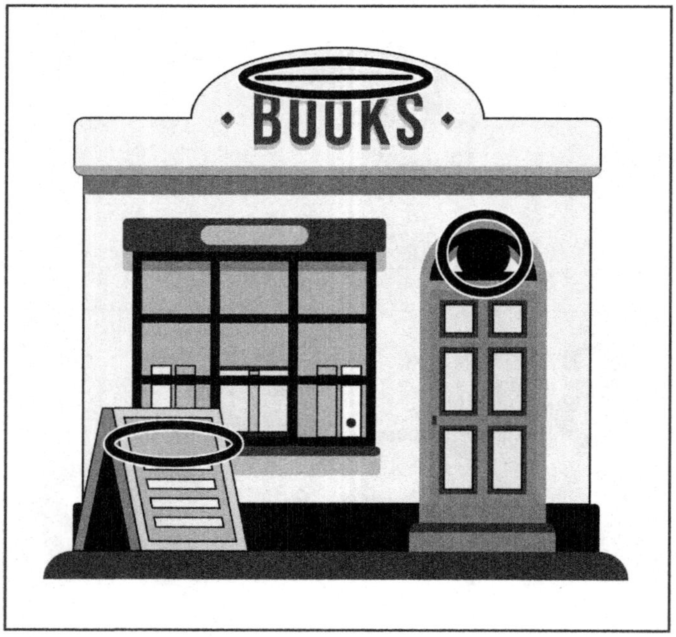

Page 53: Find 3 Differences

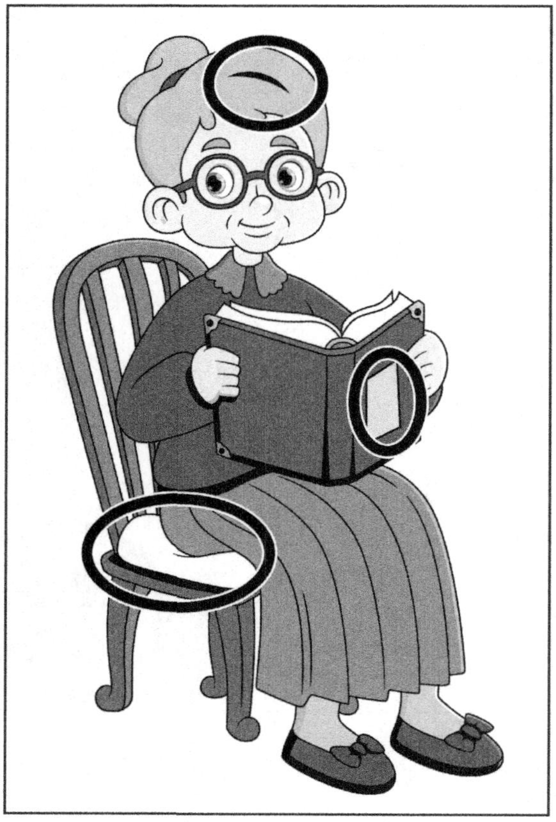

Page 54: Find 3 Differences

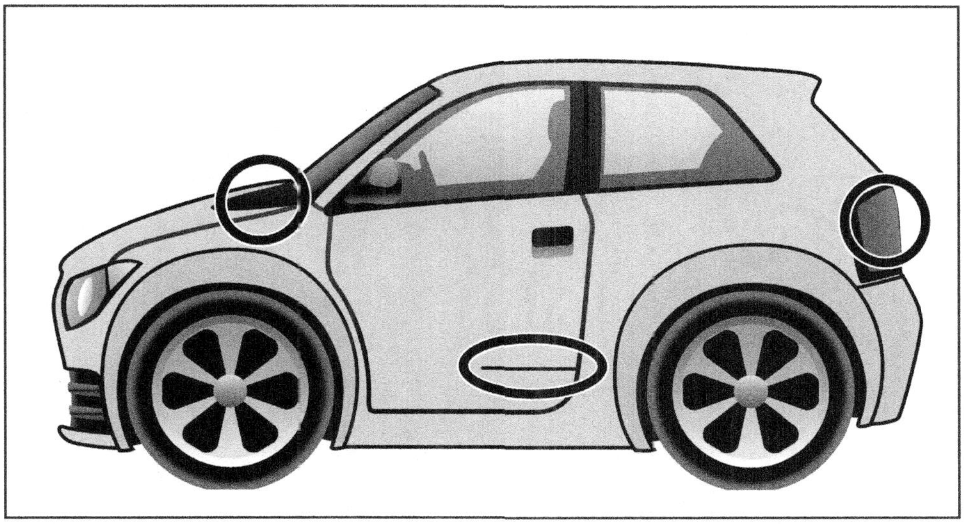

Page 56: Find 3 Differences

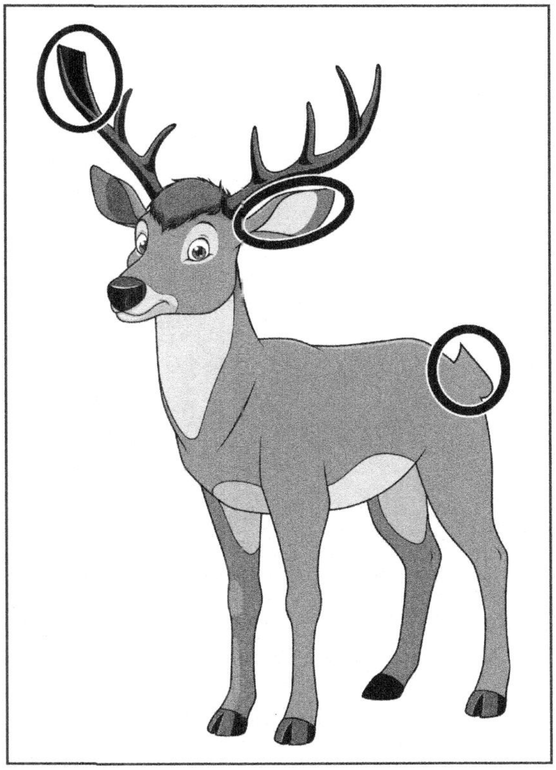

Page 55: Find 3 Differences

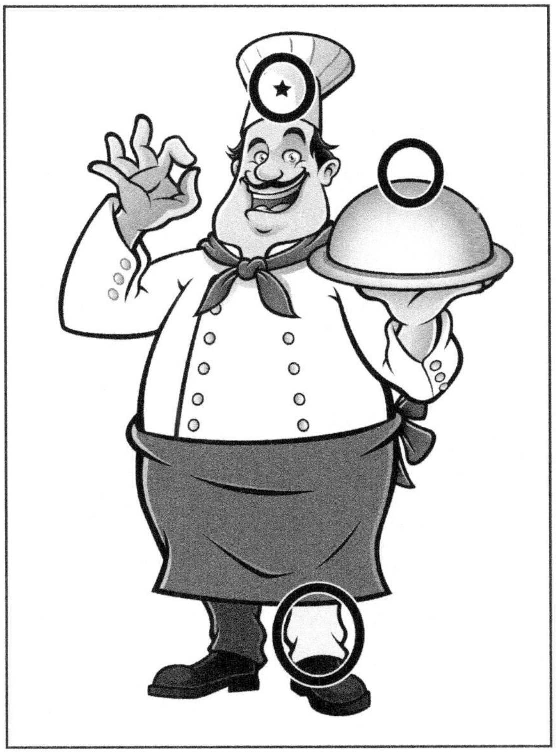

Answers

Page 57: Find 3 Differences

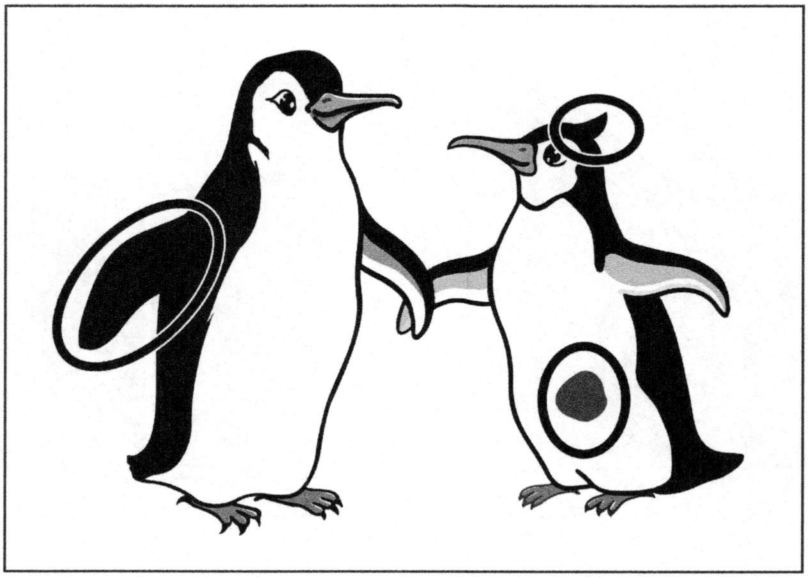

Page 58: Find 3 Differences

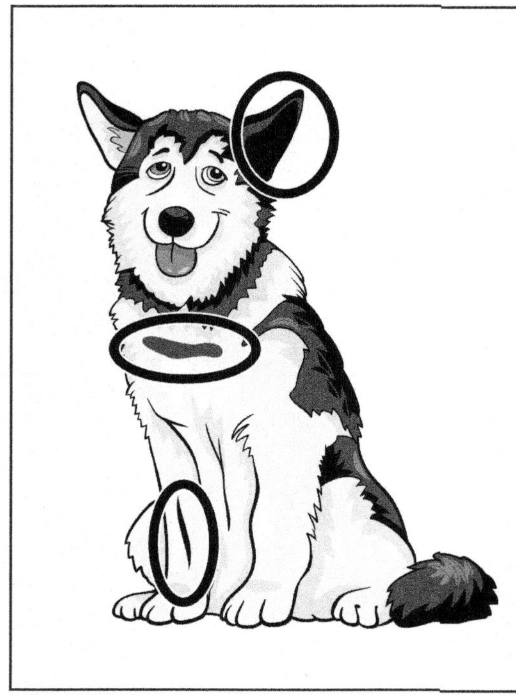

Page 59: Find 3 Differences

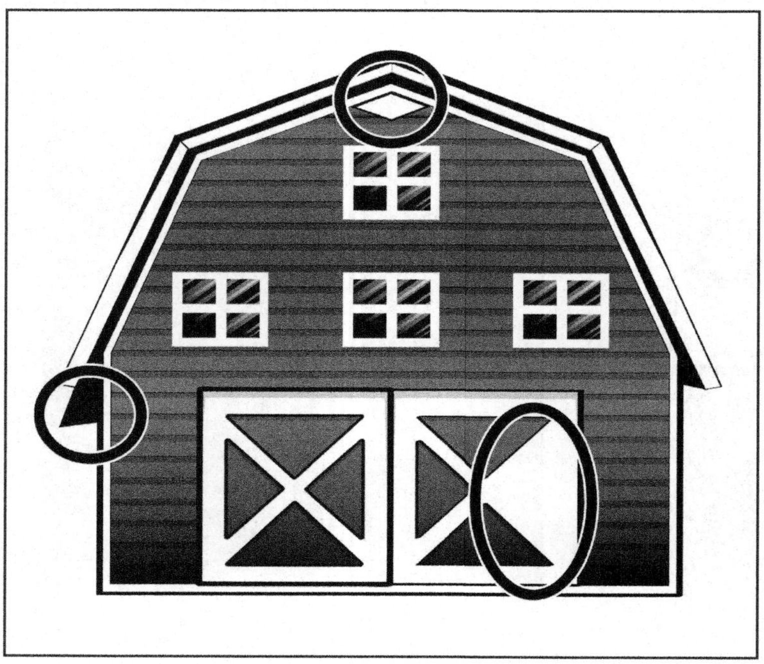

Page 60: Find 3 Differences

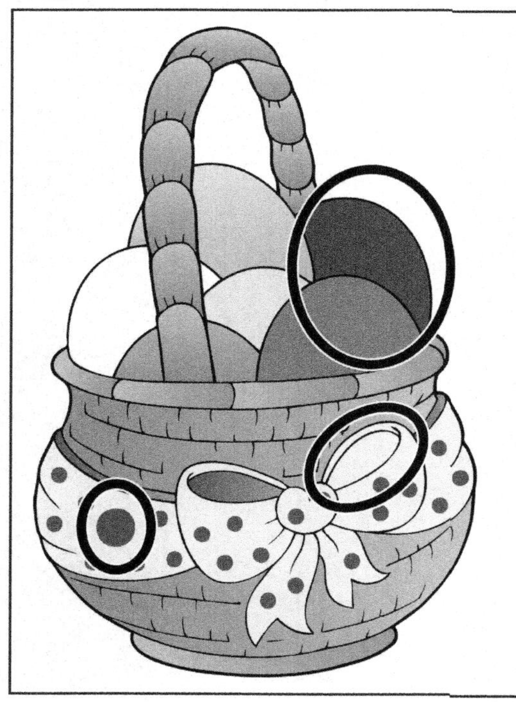

Pages 63-64: Word One

cherry sun hamburger cake mud apple

Pages 63-64: Word Two

fork plate hat cup **spoon** towel pizza

Pages 65-66: Word One

shirt glove dress sweater pie closet

Pages 65-66: Word Two

pencil bed table blanket chair book pillow **desk**

Pages 67-68: Word One

bird dog pool rabbit **house** stones forest

Pages 67-68: Word Two

rose seeds **tree** water bush sand table

Pages 69-70: Word One

paint brick cabinet t-shirt mouse **bed** fish

Pages 69-70: Word Two

window tile **milk** coat book paint yellow

Answers

Pages 71-72: Word One

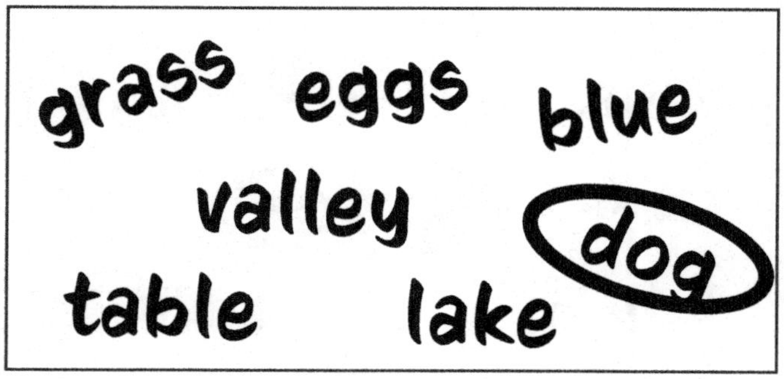

Pages 71-72: Word Two

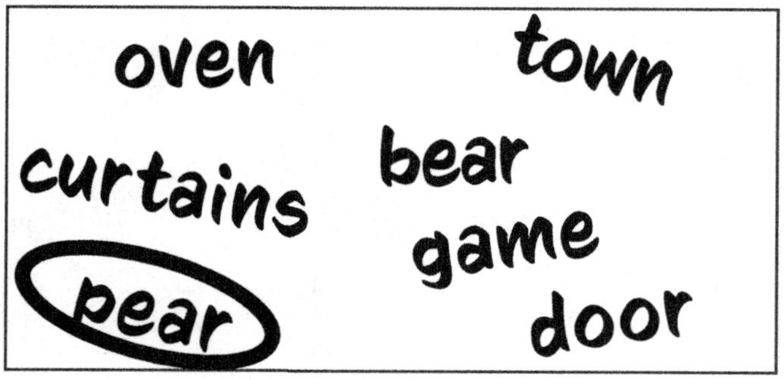

Pages 73-74: Word One

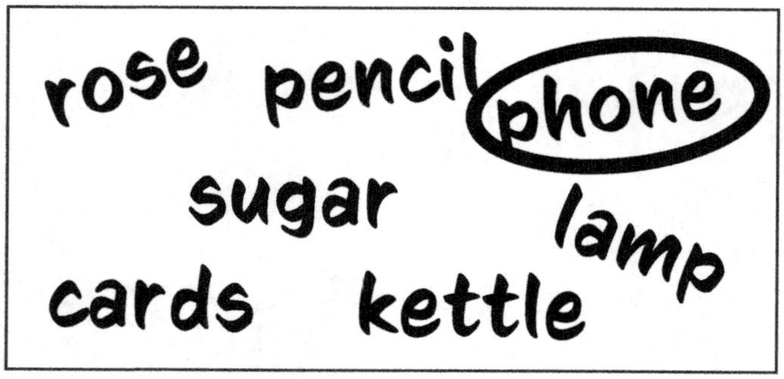

Pages 73-74: Word Two

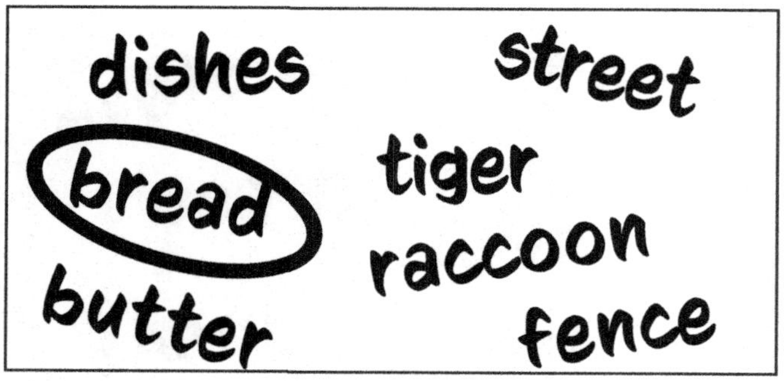

Page 77: Maze

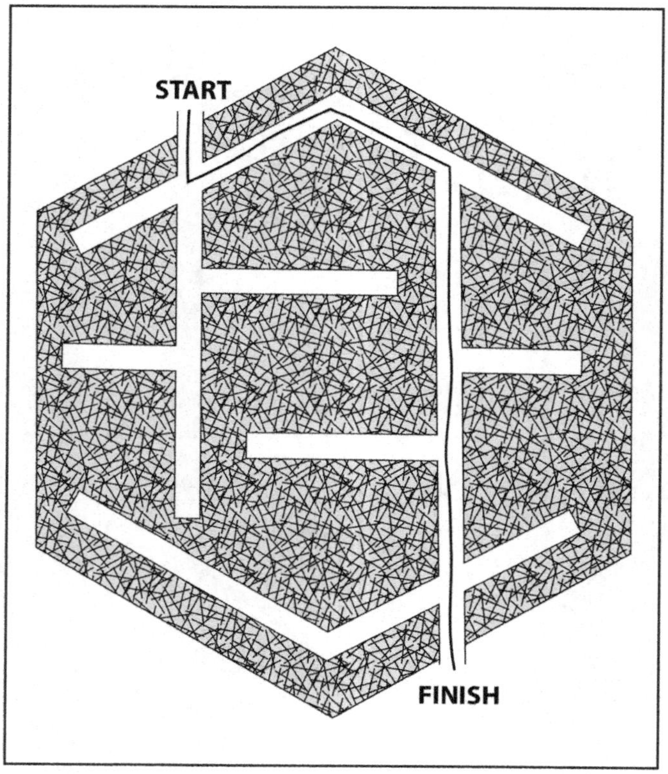

Page 78: Maze

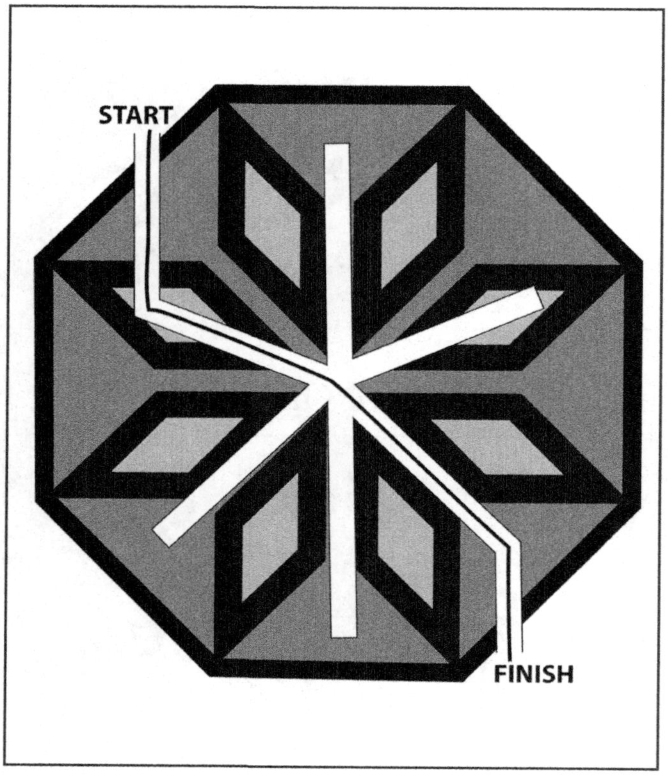

Page 79: Maze

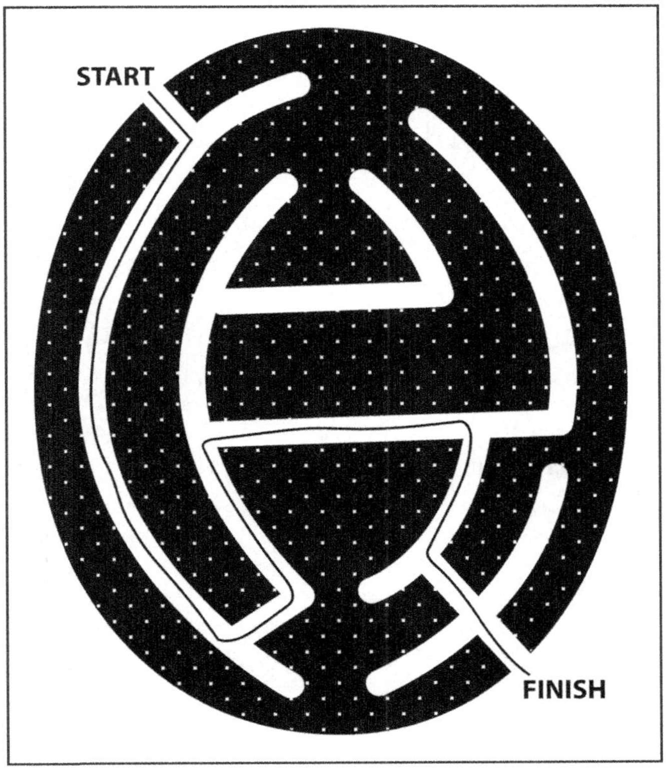

Page 80: Maze

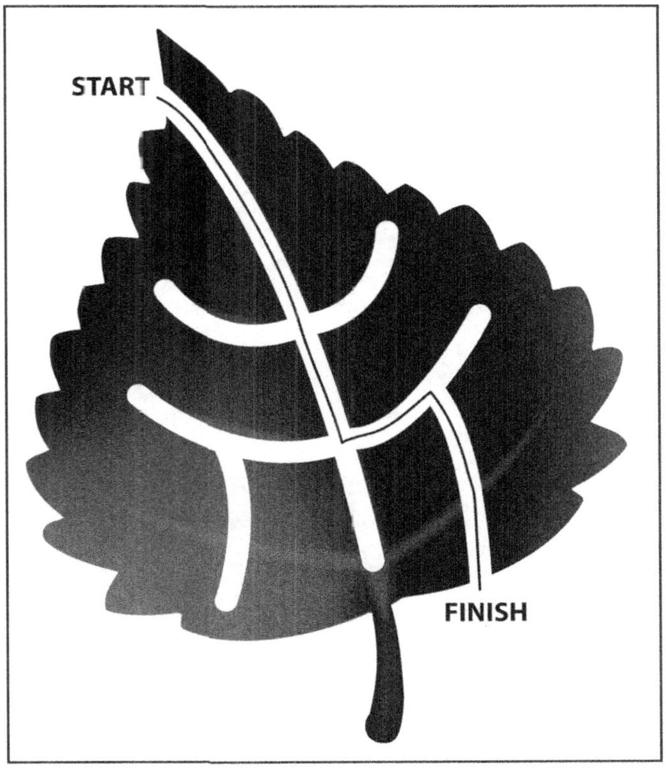

Page 81: Maze

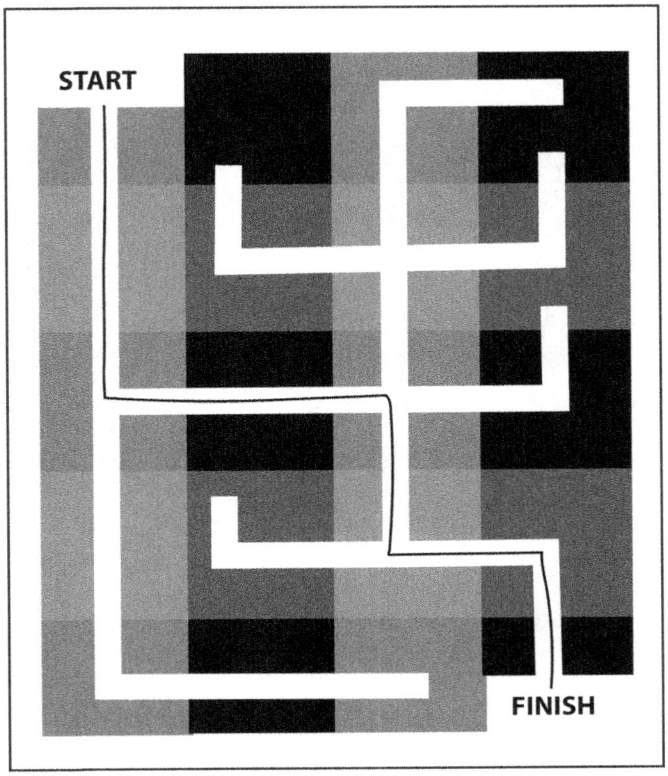

Page 82: Maze

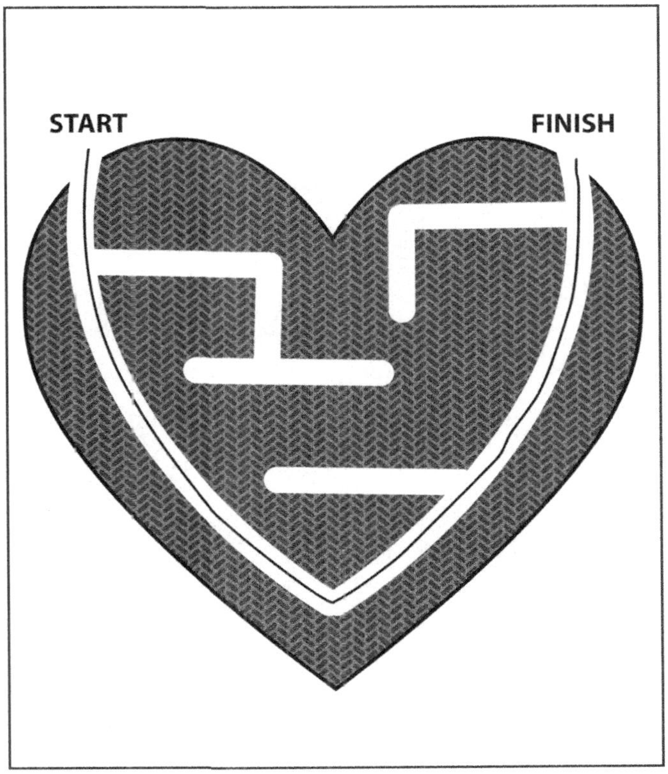

Page 83: Maze

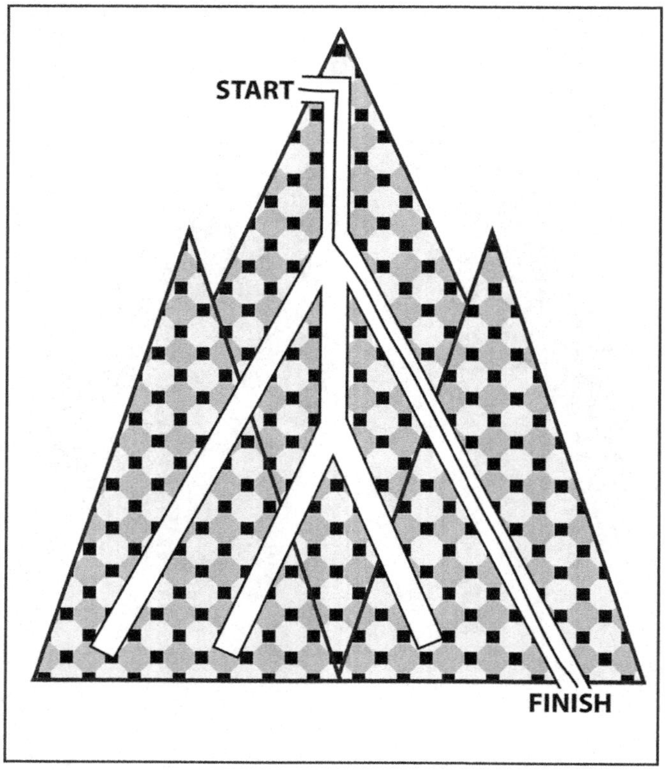

Page 84: Maze

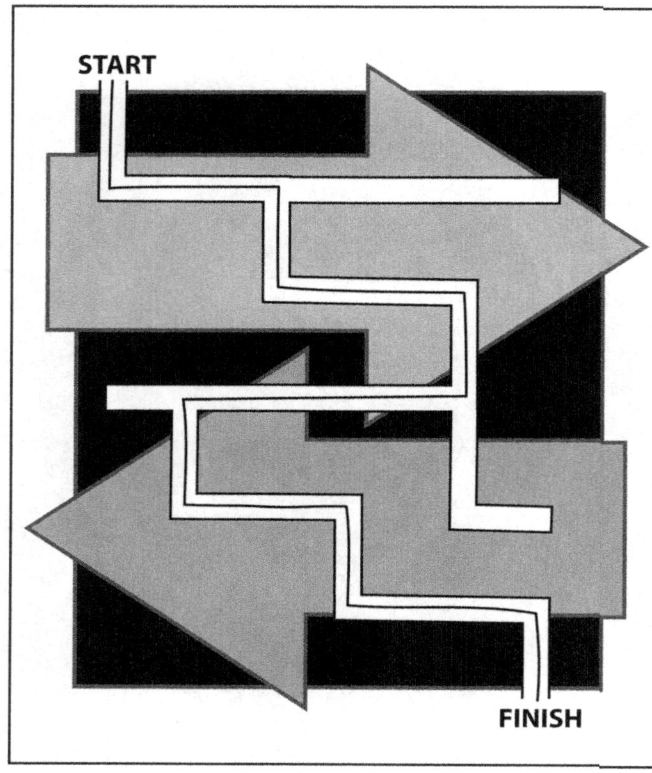

Page 85: Maze

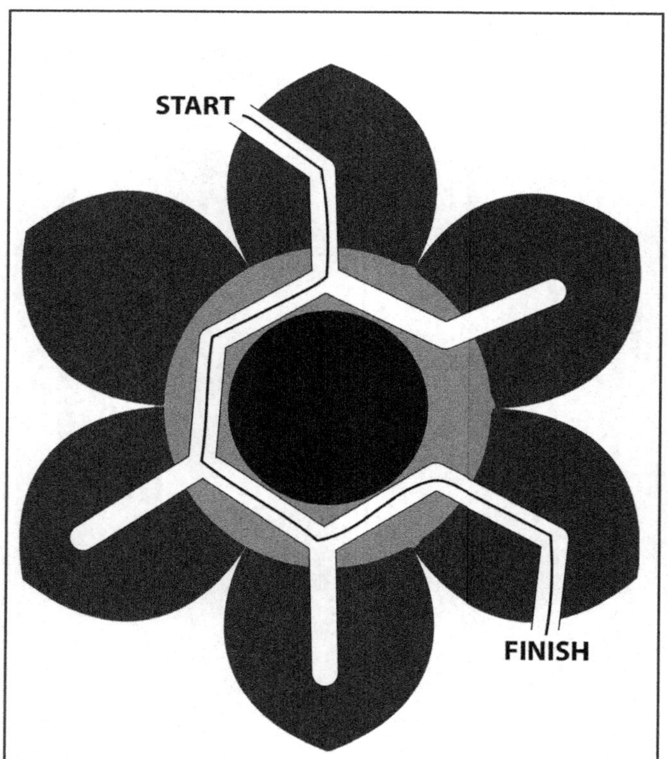

Page 86: Maze

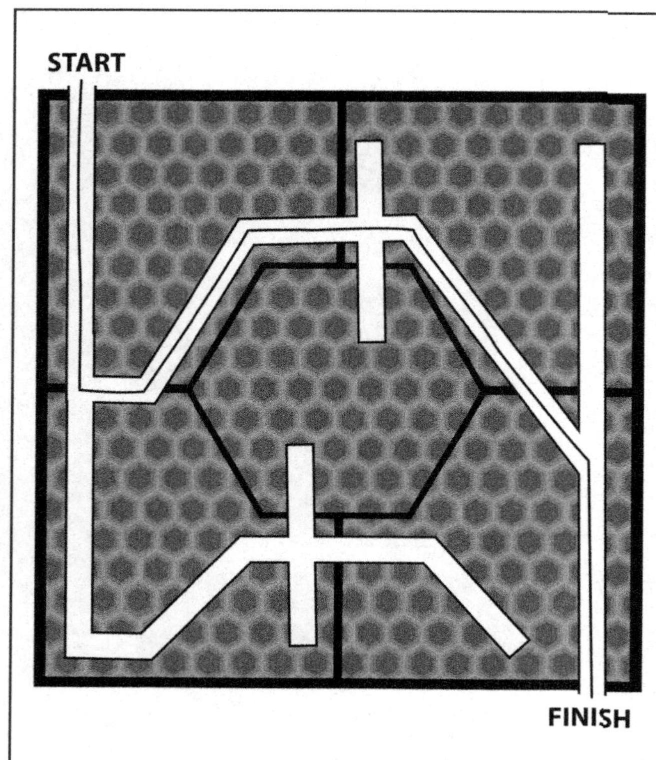

Page 87: Maze

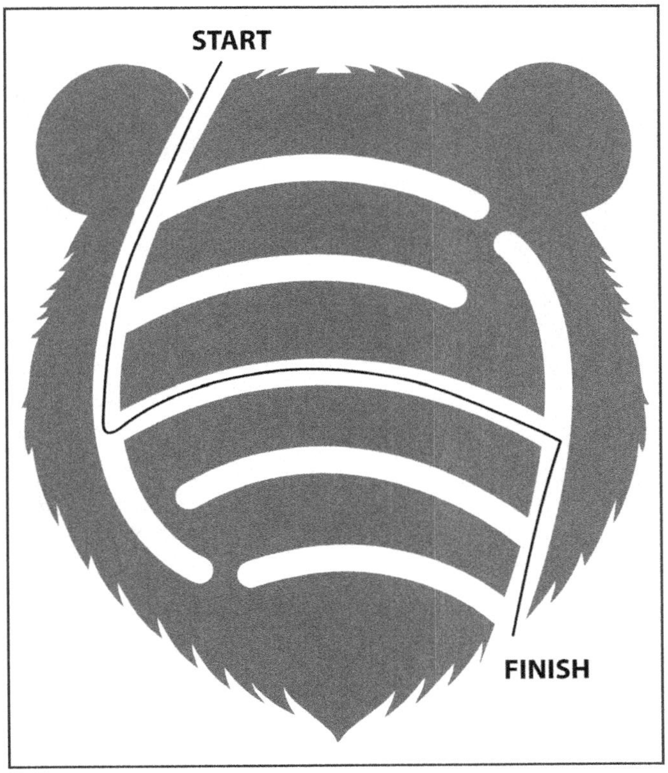

Page 88: Maze

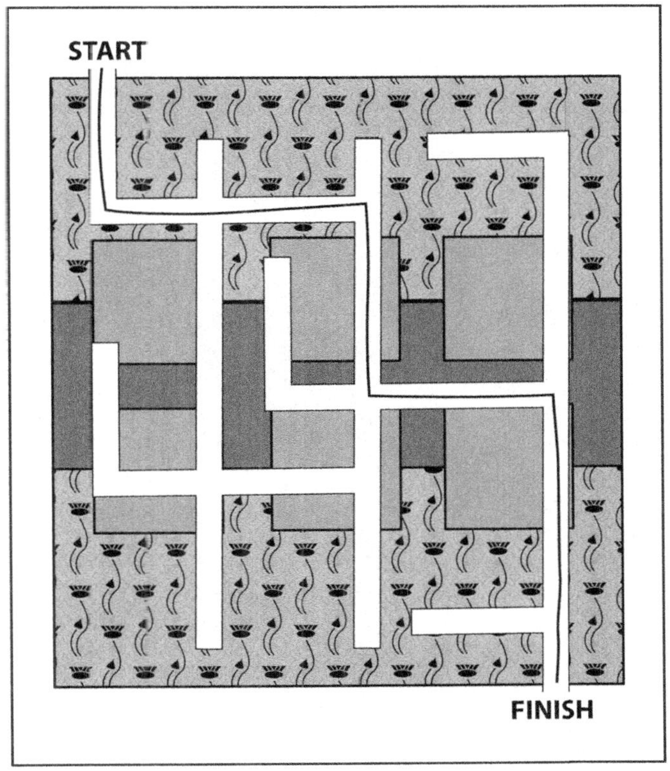

Page 90: Find 3 Differences

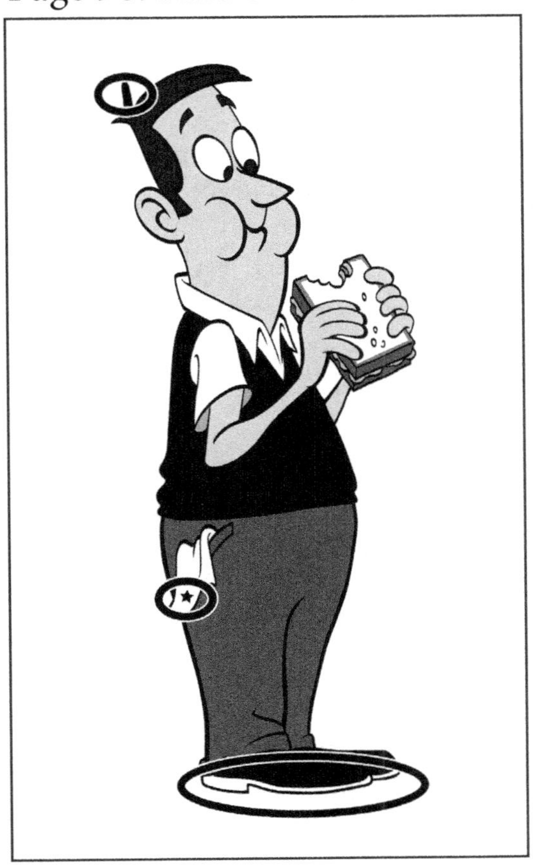

Pages 91-92 Harry's Favorite Number

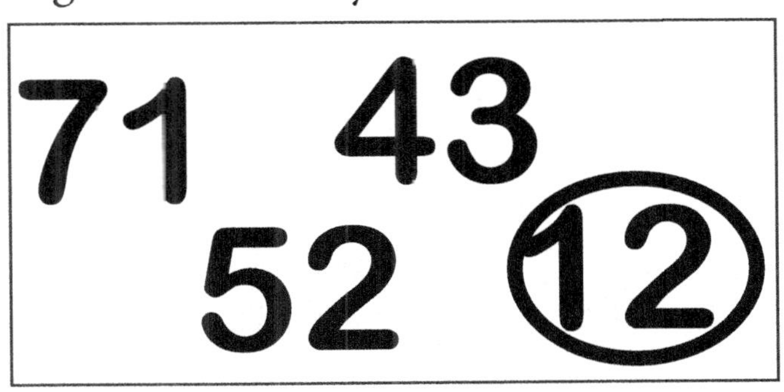

Pages 91-92: Jen's Favorite Number

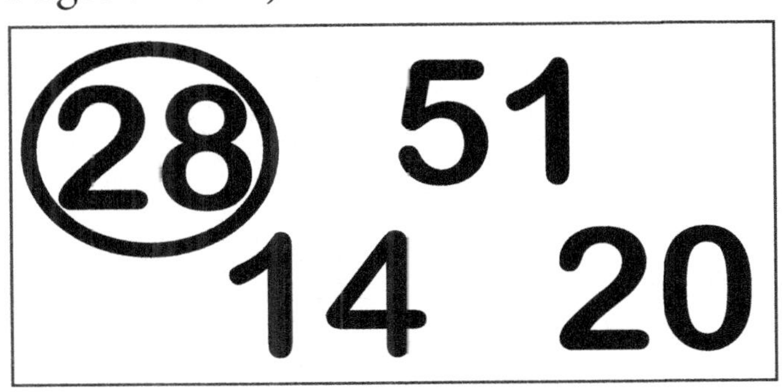

Answers

Page 93: Maze

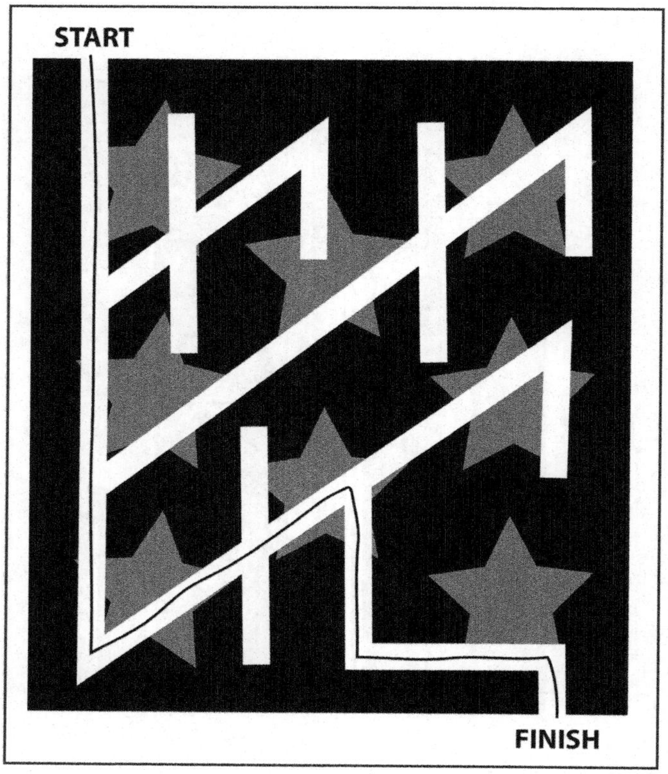

Page 94: Spot the Odd One Out

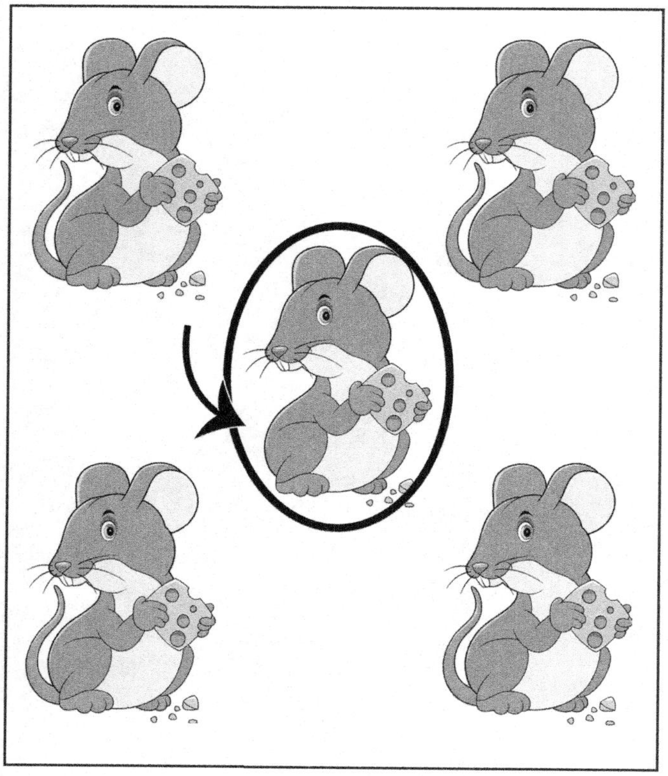

Pages 95-96: Word One

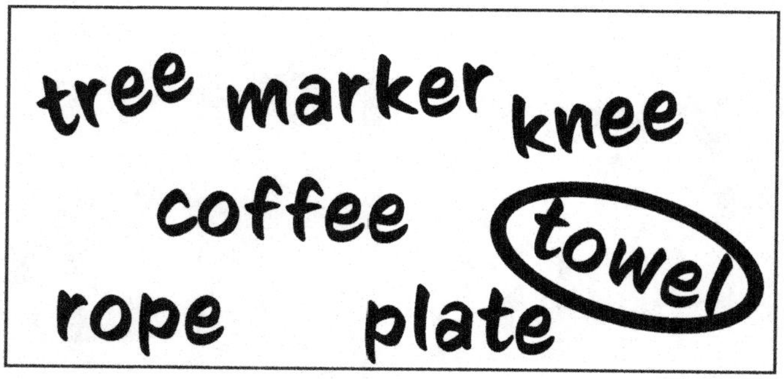

Pages 95-96: Word Two

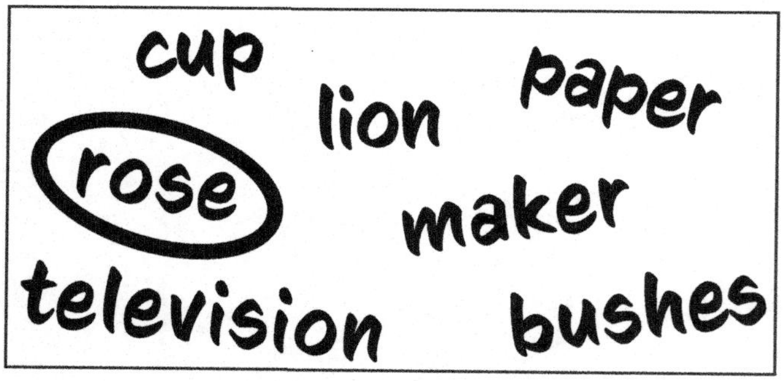

Page 97: Find the Differences

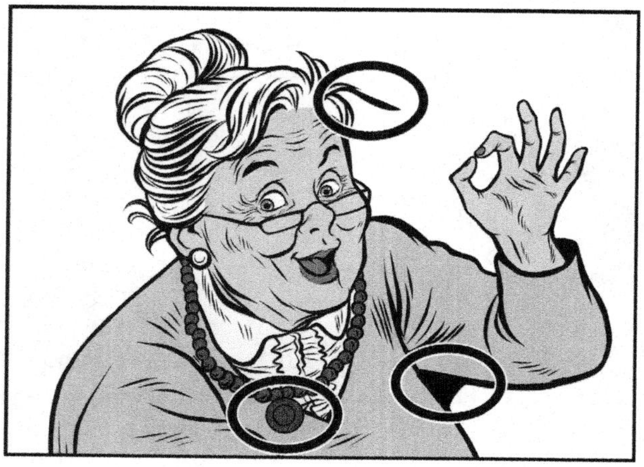

Page 98: Spot the Odd One Out

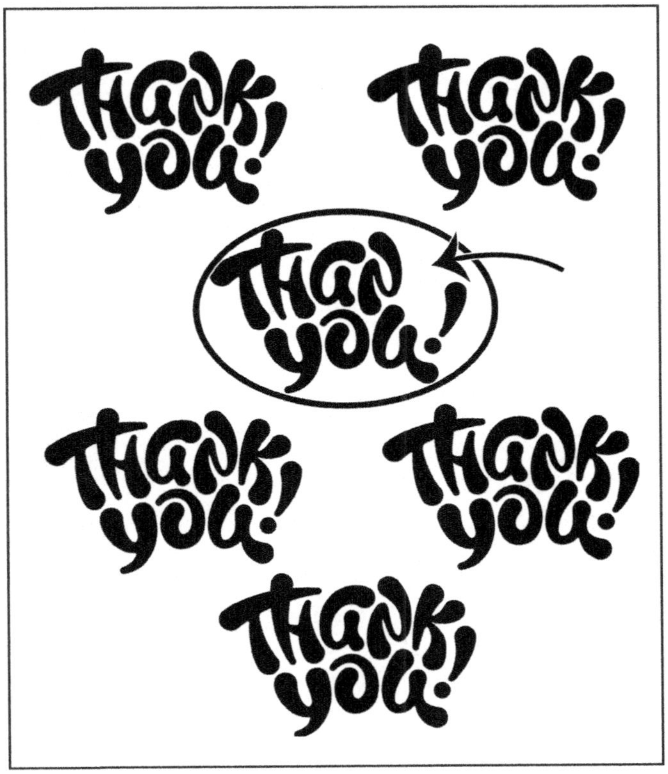

THE END

Did you enjoy this book?

Check out similar books by Joy Kinnest at:

www.LomicBooks.com

Thank you for your time!

Printed in Great Britain
by Amazon

59858203R00067